SUPPORT PARTNERS

RUN TOWARD THE ONE THEY LOVE

WHEN IN NEED, AND NOT AWAY.

THEY FEEL THE HEARTFELT PAIN

OF THE OTHER.

THEY LIFT THE OTHER UP WHEN

THEY ARE DOWN.

THEY SHARE THEIR FEARS AND

TEARS UNASHAMEDLY.

THEY WAIT AND PRAY TOGETHER WHEN

THE FUTURE IS UNKNOWN.

THEY SHARE THE MOST IMPORTANT

GIFT OF ALL,

SUPPORT—THE ABILITY TO SHARE

ONE'S OWN HEART,

EVEN WHILE IT IS BREAKING.

— JUDY KNEECE

HELPING YOUR MATE FACE

Breast Cancer

TIPS FOR BECOMING

AN EFFECTIVE

SUPPORT PARTNER

FOR THE ONE YOU LOVE

DURING THE

BREAST CANCER

EXPERIENCE

JUDY C. KNEECE, RN, OCN
BREAST HEALTH NAVIGATOR

EDUCARE INC.
3294 ASHLEY PHOSPHATE RD., SUITE 1A
N. CHARLESTON, SC 29418

Revised 6th Edition 2007; Fully Revised 5th Edition 2003; 4th Revised Edition 2001; 3rd Revised Edition 1999; 2nd Edition 1997; 1st Edition 1995.

ISBN 978-1-886665-13-2

Library of Congress Card Number: 98-93958

Printed in the United States of America

Published by EduCare Publishing Inc.

To order:

    EduCare Inc.

    3294 Ashley Phosphate Road, Suite 1A

    North Charleston, S.C. 29418

    843-760-6064 or Fax: 843-760-6988

    www.BreastHealthCare.com

Publisher's Cataloging-in-Publication

Kneece, Judy C.

Helping your mate face breast cancer: tips for becoming an effective support partner for the one you love during the breast cancer experience / Judy C. Kneece. — 6th ed.

    p. cm.

    Includes bibliographical references and index.

    ISBN: 978-1-886665-13-2

    Preassigned LCCN: 99-93958

    1. Breast—Cancer—Patients. 2. Cancer—Patients—Family relationships. I. Title.

RC280.B8K64 2003   616.99'449

                              QBI01-121

DEDICATION

This book is dedicated to all the patients and their mates who have shared openly and honestly about their physical and emotional journeys with breast cancer. Their courage serves as a source of inspiration and proof that facing a crisis together can make a relationship even more meaningful and fulfilling.

A special debt of gratitude is extended to Cindy Dreher, MPH, MAT, for her visionary efforts in women's health issues by recognizing the acute need for the psychosocial support of patients and their families during the breast cancer experience. It is through her personal support that I had the opportunity to develop a psychosocial program to meet this need. Her influence is evident throughout this book and in my work with breast cancer patients.

To Tom Winnett, I owe my motivation to begin programs for the support partner. After speaking to a large group of women, Tom looked at me with tears in his eyes and said, "Women have many places to go for help, but where is a man supposed to get help? . . . We hurt too." Thanks, Tom, for being frank and acting as a catalyst for including the support partner and family in all of my work as a breast health navigator.

From Tom's expressed need, I started a male breast cancer support group. My final dedication is to all of these support partners who have shared openly with me their fears, emotional pain, challenges and triumphs experienced in their new role. This book reflects their journey as retold to me as their breast cancer navigator. Without a doubt, I can say that an effective supportive partner is as needed as any medical treatment we can provide for a newly diagnosed breast cancer patient.

ACKNOWLEDGMENTS

A special word of appreciation to the following people for their contributions to this work:

Edward P. Dalton, M.D., F.A.C.S., and *Brian Gelfand,M.D., F.A.C.S.*, Dedicated Breast Surgeons, Elliot Hospital Breast Center, Manchester, New Hampshire, for their surgical review and clinical input.

Maurice Nahabedian, M.D., F.A.C.S., Director, Center for Reconstructive Surgery, Johns Hopkins Medical Institutions for review of the reconstruction information.

Ervin Shaw, M.D., Pathologist, Lexington Medical Center, West Columbia, South Carolina, for reviewing the pathology section.

Marianna Maldonado, M.D., Columbia, South Carolina, Psychiatrist and breast cancer survivor, for her insightful expertise in the psychological recovery from breast cancer.

Randi Rosenberg, President, Young Survival Coalition for manuscript review.

Cindy Dreher, MPH, MAT, for her support, encouragement and valuable input concerning the psychosocial issues of the breast cancer experience.

Reverend Sinclair Lewis, M.Div., D.D., Methodist pastor, and *Betty Lewis*, breast cancer survivor, for their manuscript review.

Al Barrineau and *Brian Cluxton*, support partners, for their commentaries on their experiences during their mate's breast cancer.

Debra Strange, Art Illustrations

TABLE OF CONTENTS

ABOUT THE AUTHOR

Judy C. Kneece, RN, OCN, is a certified oncology nurse with a specialty in breast cancer and is a MammaCare® Specialist, as well as an author, trainer, and consultant. She presently serves as a national Breast Health Consultant for hospitals and breast centers on the educational and psychosocial needs of the breast patient. She conducts strategic planning and oversees implementation of a comprehensive program of education and support for patients and trains nurses in a forty-hour training course to fill the role of breast health educator.

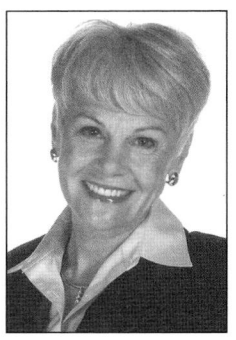

Judy is the author of five books, 41 national journal articles, 356 Patient Education Teaching Topics, *The Breast Health Navigator Manual* and *The Breast Center Strategic Planning Guide*. Her books, *Your Breast Cancer Treatment Handbook, Helping Your Mate Face Breast Cancer* and *Finding a Lump In Your Breast*, have all received outstanding reviews in the Journal of the National Cancer Institute. She is also the author of *Solving the Mystery of Breast Pain* and *Solving the Mystery of Breast Discharge*. She is a contributing editor to major women's magazine articles about breast health, including *Redbook, Marie Claire, Self, Good Housekeeping, Women's Day* and others.

EduCare's Internet site (www.educareinc.com), launched in 1995, was one of the first breast health sites on the web and presently serves approximately 200,000 people per month.

Judy has led efforts in the past several years to research the topics of recurrent breast cancer and its psychological and social impact and, most recently, sexuality issues after chemotherapy. To gather the information, focus groups of survivors were convened across the nation. Data from these focus groups was collected utilizing interactive computers. The final studies have detailed the experience of these survivors and identified their needs for education and support.

As an instructor, Judy has trained and certified over 1,500 nurses internationally in a forty-hour training course on how to implement programs of education and support for breast health patients in breast centers. In the last fourteen years she has led an international effort to change the care-delivery of breast cancer patients by (1) identifying breast cancer patient's needs through focus groups, interviews and surveys; (2) instructing nurses on how to deliver patient-focused care in a forty-hour breast health navigator certification program; and (3) leading strategic planning workshops for hospitals to teach how to implement a comprehensive breast care program that includes the psychosocial needs of women.

Judy served as a member of the National Consortium of Breast Centers' board of directors for eight years and as the editor of its newsletter, the *Breast Center Bulletin*. She recently served as a guest expert for the American Cancer Society's planning and taping of a new recurrent video series. She presently serves as a member of the Department of Defense Breast Health Scientific Advisory Board representing the interests of breast health patients in the area of educational and psychosocial needs.

As a regular conference speaker and trainer, Judy is best known for her advocacy of the breast cancer patient's psychological and social needs.

THE VOICES OF EXPERIENCE:

When I finished writing this manuscript, it was not really complete. It lacked the voice of experience—a peer who had actually lived through the experience. You, a new support partner, needed to hear from someone who had personally experienced the same feelings, fears, challenges, and joys of the support role you have inherited. My experience has been as a coach for couples, offering professional support by helping them to identify the challenges ahead and how to develop skills to best deal with them. I have not actually experienced the role of being a support partner to a mate during a breast cancer diagnosis. To offer you the experience of a peer, I have asked two mates to share their perspective of the support partner experience on a variety of topics.

Sprinkled throughout this book are their feelings about the intimate experiences they faced during their support partner role. It is our hope that the sharing of their personal journey will give you the courage to know that you and the one you love are not alone. Others have faced the same challenges and managed to face this unexpected life crisis, using it as a time to grow closer emotionally. It is not an easy process, but it is achievable. I want to introduce you to two support partners, Al Barrineau and Brian Cluxton.

AL BARRINEAU
SUPPORT PARTNER

I had the privilege of working with Al and his wife, Harriett, for three years in the early 1990's, as they worked through the breast cancer experience. Involved with them in their journey were four sons, who were then ages 14 to 21.

Harriett was diagnosed with a large tumor that required a mastectomy. Eventually, she underwent a second mastectomy and bilateral reconstruction. During this time they were active in support groups, sharing their pain during their journey and offering encouragement to others. Harriett has served as a reach to recovery volunteer, and they both remained active in support groups for several years.

Al has shared his challenges and struggles with many other spouses. Throughout this book he reveals many of his feelings and experiences with you. Harriett provides the same commentary for the patient's book, *Your Breast Cancer Treatment Handbook.*

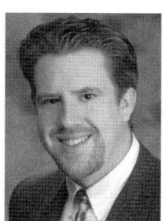

BRIAN CLUXTON
SUPPORT PARTNER

Brian was starting the phase of his life that most men look forward to—settling down with the girl of his dreams. He was getting married.

The wedding went off without a hitch. They went to Jamaica for their honeymoon. His wife shared with him that she could feel a lump under a flat area of the skin on her breast. When they arrived home as a new couple, she called her OB/GYN who decided to perform an ultrasound and immediately decided a mammogram was also needed. She had a surgical consult with a fine needle biopsy seven days after they had been sitting on a beach in Jamaica. Twenty minutes after the biopsy, they heard the words, "Well, it looks positive for cancer." Brian recalls, "We were completely flattened by the news. I can't even remember what else the doctor said to us after those words."

One month after the wedding, Anna underwent seven hours of surgery for a mastectomy with an immediate TRAM flap reconstruction. All 16 lymph nodes removed from surgery came back negative. Anna had chemotherapy. The day of her first chemo treatment, Brian shaved his head to show his support. "When other couples are starting out their new life together, I was sitting on the bathroom floor holding Anna as she was throwing up."

Brian reflects, "She was young, too young for breast cancer some would think. But breast cancer does happen to young women. . . . Cancer has changed our lives as individuals and as a couple. Anna is now active in the Young Survival Coalition, which educates and supports young people with breast cancer. She works for breast health services at the same hospital where she received her treatment. Daily she interacts with other women hearing the same words we heard—the biopsy is positive for cancer."

Anna and Brian's life changed quickly. They were a very young couple facing a breast cancer diagnosis, but they have allowed an unexpected visitor to turn their lives into a mission to help others. I asked Brian to share how a young support partner thinks and responds to the different decisions that have to be made. Throughout this book you will read Brian's response to Anna's cancer diagnosis as a young newlywed and a support partner. Anna provides the same commentary for the patient's book, *Your Breast Cancer Treatment Handbook*.

15

PERSPECTIVE

"WE GAIN PERSPECTIVE BY

HAVING SOMEONE AT OUR SIDE.

WE GAIN OBJECTIVITY.

WE GAIN COURAGE IN

THREATENING SITUATIONS.

HAVING OTHERS NEAR

TEMPERS OUR DOGMATISM AND

SOFTENS OUR INTOLERANCE.

WE GAIN ANOTHER OPINION.

WE GAIN WHAT TODAY

IS CALLED INPUT."

— CHUCK SWINDOLL

INTRODUCTION TO THE SUPPORT ROLE

> *'I'm sorry; the tumor is malignant. Your wife has breast cancer.' Those few words sent a chill through me. Those words would test all human emotion in me during the weeks and months to come.*
>
> **—AL BARRINEAU**
> **SUPPORT PARTNER**

Cancer. This is one of the most terrifying words in the English language. When you hear it applied to someone you love, its meaning amplifies and grows to paralyzing proportions. Shock, fear, confusion, and denial may absorb your mind and body. There is no "Cancer 101" training to prepare you to know what to do or say, where to go for help, or how to be the most supportive partner to the one you love. You have inherited a new role—support partner. This is a role with many new demands.

A breast cancer diagnosis stresses and shakes the equilibrium of a relationship. Dr. Marilyn T. Oberst sums up the stress placed on those who inherit a support role:

> *"Learning to live with cancer is clearly no easy task. Learning to live with someone else's cancer may be even more **difficult**, precisely because no one recognizes just how **hard** it really is to **deal** with **someone else's cancer."***

Living with someone else's cancer is a challenge; but it is one which can be mastered successfully. The key is to learn how to manage and balance the emotional and physical demands.

Many examples quoted in this book are from the most common support partner, a spouse. However, the same principles of support apply to anyone who serves as the primary support person for a breast cancer patient. Often this may be a parent, sibling, or a friend serving in this role.

This book was written from my experience working with and observing hundreds of breast cancer patients and their support partners as they lived through the cancer experience. My work allowed me to maintain an ongoing relationship with the patient and her partner throughout the course of her treatment and recovery. My goal is to help you understand the challenge of living with the pain of someone else's breast cancer diagnosis, and to assist you in becoming a more effective support person.

> *We were both frozen in fear after we heard the word cancer. I don't remember anything else the doctor said after this. I was emotionally stunned.*
>
> —BRIAN CLUXTON
> SUPPORT PARTNER

Many patients and their support partners have openly shared with me their pain and efforts to make "sense out of a senseless situation" in hopes that the breast cancer experience will be more positive for those like you who inherit the role. I once heard, "If you want to find your way out of a forest, it is not as helpful to ask a forester, who knows all about the trees, but to ask someone who was lost but managed to find the way out of the forest." This book is from those who managed to find their own way through the forest of the breast cancer experience.

This book is not designed as a comprehensive manual on coping. Instead, it is a combination of life experiences from patients, their support partners, and my clinical experience. I urge you to reach out to other professionals—counselors, physicians, nurses and support groups—to complete your understanding of the "support" role.

Through this book you will also gain an understanding of the basics of the breast cancer treatment process. You will learn effective and supportive techniques to ease the process, and you will find additional resources available to assist you and your family. The support role is not an easy one, but it is one from which you can learn and grow as you provide one of the most powerful tools for your mate's recovery from breast cancer—effective support.

My best wishes for a rewarding support experience,

Judy

WHAT IS A SUPPORT PARTNER?

> *My wife has always been the caretaker and care giver in our family. She nursed us during illness, praised our accomplishments, encouraged us in our trials, paid the compliments, initiated the hugging—now the roles were reversed. She needed these things from me. My world had been shaken to the core. I wasn't sure I could be what she needed.*
>
> **—AL BARRINEAU**
> **SUPPORT PARTNER**

You have inherited a new role: support partner for a breast cancer patient. What does the role of support partner mean? It is best described by the *American Heritage Dictionary* (Fourth Edition).

support v. 1. To bear the weight of, especially from below. 2. To hold in position so as to keep from falling, sinking, or slipping. 3. To be capable of bearing; withstand. 4. To keep from weakening or failing; strengthen. 5. To provide for or maintain, by supplying with money or necessities. 6. To furnish corroborating evidence for. 7. To aid the cause, policy, or interests of. 8. To endure; tolerate. 9. To act in a secondary or subordinate role to (a leading performer).

support n. 1. a. The act of supporting. b. The state of being supported. 2. One that supports. 3. Maintenance, as of a family, with the necessities of life.

partner n. 1. One that is united or associated with another or others in an activity or a sphere of common interest. a. A spouse.

A support partner is someone who helps you maintain your balance during a crisis; someone bound to another by a relationship, commitment, or a common bond of interest. Support partners stand alongside the ones they love as a stabilizing force, sharing the emotional and physical burden. The role is a subordinate role, in that the patient takes the lead role in making decisions and sets the emotional tone.

We were newlyweds. I was just learning to become a husband when I was cast into the role of support partner for my wife with breast cancer. To say I was overwhelmed in my ability to meet this new challenge was an understatement.

—BRIAN CLUXTON
SUPPORT PARTNER

However, the support partner is the one who provides the fertile environment of caring, who assists in information gathering, fosters hope and assures the partner of their commitment for the duration of the crisis. The role of support partner is as important as any medical treatment the patient will receive. The gift of your support can make the difference in her physical and emotional recovery.

The following chapters include ways others have successfully filled this role. I challenge you to learn from those who have shared and to add your own inventive methods of support. I wish you a very rewarding support-role experience.

REMEMBER

YOUR ROLE AS A

SUPPORT PARTNER

IS ONE OF THE

MOST IMPORTANT

COMPONENTS FOR

THE EMOTIONAL

RECOVERY

OF THE

ONE YOU LOVE.

CHAPTER 2

THE INITIAL DIAGNOSIS

"Y ou have breast cancer" are four words that forever change lives. The patient and those closest to her are suddenly faced with an unexpected challenge. Unplanned. Unprepared. Helpless. Confused. These are the terms that best describe the diagnostic period. Yet, in the midst of all the emotions is the urgent need to make critical decisions about treatment. Most patients and their support partners are ill-prepared for the decisions they are required to make about future healthcare decisions. There is no course in Breast Cancer 101 to prepare for this life experience. Most are thrust into the experience unexpectedly and forced to learn quickly about decisions that have lifetime effects.

If you are feeling overwhelmed emotionally and physically about the tasks that lay ahead of both of you, you are normal. Most people feel intensely ill-prepared and afraid of what the future holds. Understanding the emotions involved in a breast cancer diagnosis is as important as understanding the physical treatments. The healthcare team is prepared to take care of the physical components—surgery, radiation, and chemotherapy treatments. However, most patients and their support partners are left to find their own way through the emotional maze in which they find themselves.

> When Anna went for a breast biopsy, I thought it would just be a cyst like her mother had had. The biopsy was no big deal; besides, it was so simple it was being done as an outpatient procedure. Anna was only 32; too young for cancer. When her pathology report can back with the diagnosis of "cancer," I went into emotional shock that lasted for days. It had never occurred to me that it would be cancer. I could not sleep at all the first few days. My mind kept torturing me with the fact that Anna could die and I would be a widower at 28.

—BRIAN CLUXTON
SUPPORT PARTNER

21

Shock and fear best describe my first reaction. This was only supposed to happen to other women—not my wife. We were both in a daze. But one thing was for sure; my wife and I were in this together from the start.

—AL BARRINEAU
SUPPORT PARTNER

Understanding the emotional aspects of a diagnosis is essential, and understanding the actions that can help manage the crisis that suddenly turns your life upside down is equally important. This is the purpose of this book: helping you to understand how to best help yourself and your partner by understanding and recommending ways to cope with and prevent problems.

EMOTIONAL ADJUSTMENT

The time from diagnosis through surgery is an acute phase of adjustment for the patient, partner, and family members. During this time you and your partner will be required to learn about the disease and its treatments, emotions, and effective communication skills. Your goal is to successfully maneuver through the experience and emerge emotionally intact. How this is accomplished will differ, based on your personality, the personality of the patient, and both of your previous problem solving and coping experiences. Even though relationship dynamics may be different, many problems and their solutions are common for the patient and for you, the support person.

During an unexpected crisis, there are some general physical and emotional changes that may occur in you or your mate. It is helpful to know that these symptoms are all signs of stress.

Changes that you or your mate may experience:

- **Body**—headaches, feelings of exhaustion, stomach problems, minor pains, decreased resistance to colds, flu, etc.
- **Mind**—negative thoughts, confusion, difficulty concentrating, sleeplessness, forgetting details, mind going blank, lower productivity
- **Feelings**—anxiety, anger, fear, frustration, emotional withdrawal

You or your partner may experience these symptoms of stress in varying degrees. They are not a result of illness, but of a natural emotional reaction affecting the physical body during a crisis. Awareness of the symptoms and monitored rest are needed. If they become severe or unmanageable, contact your healthcare provider. They are there to help you, but they can only do so when you let them know your needs. However, one of the most effective strategies for managing these symptoms is support. Your support for your loved one and the support you seek for yourself will reduce the stress of the crisis. Support is a buffer against stress and a very important factor during a crisis.

REMEMBER

A CRISIS MAY CAUSE PHYSICAL AS WELL AS MENTAL CHANGES.

SEEK THE ADVICE OF YOUR HEALTHCARE TEAM IF THE SYMPTOMS BECOME UNMANAGEABLE.

SUPPORT PARTNERS

LET THEIR PARTNER:
BORROW THEIR SHOULDERS
WHEN THEY NEED
A PLACE TO LEAN;

BORROW THEIR EYES
WHEN THEIRS ARE
FILLED WITH TEARS;

BORROW THEIR HEART
WHEN THEIRS IS BROKEN;

BORROW THEIR STRENGTH
WHEN THEY ARE WEAK;

BORROW THEIR FAITH
WHEN THEIRS IS SHAKEN;

BORROW THEIR SUPPORT WHEN
ALL OTHERS DESERT THEM.

— JUDY KNEECE

DEALING WITH YOUR OWN EMOTIONAL PAIN

At the time of diagnosis, all attention from the medical staff, family members and friends is obviously directed toward the patient—she has breast cancer. Yet, as a support partner, it is also a very difficult and painful time for you as the person who is closest to the patient. You may be feeling overwhelmed by expectations from yourself and others to be strong and emotionally supportive for your loved one. You may even fear others seeing you cry as you strive to remain emotionally strong. Yet, behind the emotional facade, everything in your body is crying out for relief from the unexpected emotional pain. Your heart is breaking too. It is very important for her emotional recovery, as well as your own, that you recognize your pain as normal and take steps to have your own needs met. At this time, just as she needs a support network, you also need a support system to help you understand your new role as support partner.

Support partners suffer emotions similiar to the one who is diagnosed, because of the intimate emotional and physical attachment shared. You may be surprised to find that you experience and mirror many of the same emotions as your partner—shock, numbness, disbelief, confusion, anger, and sadness. While you may express your emotions differently because of your personality, the underlying emotion is the same. Remember, some people will strike out at others when angry, while others may withdraw from the person at which they are angry. The underlying emotion is the same even though the response is different. The important thing to remember is

> *My heart was broken, yet I was afraid to let Anna see me cry. I didn't want to upset her anymore than she was already. However one day, my emotions became so overwhelming that I finally broke down and cried in front of her. To my surprise, it was very helpful and comforting to both of us.*
>
> **—BRIAN CLUXTON**
> **SUPPORT PARTNER**

that you will find yourself experiencing many emotions, some that may be new to you. It is important to remember that it is normal during the crisis of a partner's diagnosis to experience a wide range of emotions. You have also been forced to embrace a dreaded enemy.

This is a sad time for both of you. Grieving is a natural and helpful way for healing to begin. Many find it difficult to openly express these feelings of grief to others for fear that they may appear "weak" or "not in control." The opposite is true. These feelings show that you are very much attuned to what is occurring in your life. Expressing feelings honestly to your partner will not weaken your relationship but will strengthen it. Expressing your feelings to others helps reduce the intensity of an emotion.

> *I needed to come to grips with the cancer. I thought the word cancer was an automatic death sentence. I was overwhelmed with the decisions we faced, the quick education we had to get about cancer. At the same time, I appreciated that my wife included me in the process.*
>
> **—AL BARRINEAU**
> **SUPPORT PARTNER**

Ann Kaiser Sterns summed up the scary feeling grief causes when she said, "The experience of grief is not mental illness—it just feels that way sometimes." At times you may feel a complete loss of control over life as you once knew it. At times you may feel as if you are "losing it mentally." This feeling is common, and is a part of working through a new life crisis.

HOLDING BACK EMOTIONS

Many support partners try to hold back their deep emotional pain and avoid crying. This is not helpful to you or to your partner. Tears do not signal a "loss of control" but are more likely to convey the intimate love you have for her. Crying is a sign that you are dealing with your emotions in a perfectly healthy and natural way. Seeing your tears will often give her unspoken permission to share her own intense feelings and fears with you, knowing that you are very much in tune with her emotional pain.

Gregg Levoy in *Psychology Today* shares, "The amount of manganese stored in the body affects our moods, and the body stores 30 times as much manganese in tears as in blood serum. Biochemist Will Frey says 'the lacrimal gland, which determines the flow of tears, concentrates and removes manganese from the body.' Frey has also identified three other chemicals stored up by stress that are released by crying." Crying is therapeutic. After a good cry, we feel a sense of emotional release. It is similar to a rain leaving the air clear and clean when it is over. Nicholas Wolterstroff said, "Tears are salve on our wounds."

So, if you have forced yourself to be brave and hold back the tears, now is the time to emotionally free yourself and know that it is okay to cry. Tears are not a sign of weakness, but rather a sign that we are in touch with reality and are dealing with the losses that a crisis brings.

FINDING YOUR SUPPORT

As the primary support person, you will find it helpful to identify someone you can talk to who understands exactly what you are feeling. This could be a friend, family member, professional counselor or pastor. You also need a support system. You need someone to talk to that you can pour out all of your fears, anxieties and emotions, knowing that they will be there, not to be judgmental, but to offer emotional support and guidance to you personally. What often comes as a surprise is that many of the people closest to you often don't understand when you try to share. They have never had to deal with what you are going through, and they feel the best way they can help is to cheer you up, or help you get your mind off of your problems. Being cheered up and diversional activities are okay, but this is not what you need now. Every person needs at least one person to whom they can talk freely, knowing that no matter what, they will be listened to and supported. Professional counselors are skilled at crisis intervention and can identify the coping skills you already have to help you during a time like this. They can help you sort out your fears and concerns and find helpful

IT'S OKAY TO CRY

Crying is a very acceptable and healthy expression of grief.

Crying shows how deeply you feel and how much you care.

Crying helps relieve the tension that has built up inside of you.

Crying is an expression of deep contrition and unspeakable love.

Crying speaks for you when you cannot find the words.

Crying helps you to recover your physical and emotional strength.

Crying is not the mark of weakness, but of power.

Crying allows grief to be done in a constructive way.

Crying enables you to cope with a significant loss.

Crying is a way of communicating with your humanity.

Crying ventilates feelings of anger and hurt.

— ENCOURAGEMENT MINISTRIES

REMEMBER

ways to face the decisions ahead. You will find a professional counselor acts as a "safe place" to say anything you think or feel without upsetting anyone.

Cancer treatment centers often offer support services such as a partners' support group, social workers, chaplains, and counselors who are trained to help you adjust and perform in your new role of support. Call and ask your physician, nurse or social worker for a recommendation. Remember, you need support, too. You need someone who recognizes the demands placed on a support partner and who can share this experience with you and help you master your new role.

UNDERSTANDING THE IMPACT ON YOUR MATE

The diagnosis of breast cancer often confirms a woman's greatest fear. With the diagnosis she is thrown into emotional turmoil. She is faced with an array of possible losses or threats:

- loss or alteration of a breast
- loss or alteration of her previous feminine image
- threat to her sexuality and attractiveness to you as a partner
- threat to her self-esteem because of diagnosis or surgery
- threat to her future career or educational plans
- loss of her ability to maintain her functional role in the family and/or workplace during surgery or treatments
- concerns about her children and being unable to meet their future needs
- threat to her life

For a short time following diagnosis, a woman often finds herself in a state of shock and numbness as she sorts through all of these threats and potential losses. At the same time she is struggling with this, she is expected to make quick, critical decisions—decisions that require a basic knowledge of the disease and her treatment options. This usually leaves her in mental anguish, overwhelmed and with a feeling of extreme loss of control.

The most common response of newly diagnosed breast cancer patients is the underlying theme of a "loss of control." At diagnosis, they have suddenly lost control over many things in their life and are faced with a future that is unknown and filled with numerous

> *Anna was the love of my life, my new bride. All I knew was that no matter what I would be there for her. But it was important that I let her know how I viewed our future.*
>
> **—BRIAN CLUXTON**
> **SUPPORT PARTNER**

decisions. To complicate it all, these are decisions that there has been no preparation in life to deal with. They are forced—at a time in their life when anxieties are at their highest—to learn about breast cancer and treatments for it, whether they feel like it or not. As a support partner, you can greatly help restore her sense of control by understanding her emotional state and by assisting her in a manner suitable to her personality and helping her get the information she needs to make decisions.

CREATING A SAFE SPACE FOR HER EMOTIONALLY

Most women react to the diagnosis of breast cancer with intense fears and emotional withdrawal. Some find it very difficult to communicate their fears and feelings at this early time. This is all normal. Your partner needs time to grieve over the diagnosis and her loss. Now is the time to give her a "safe space" for her emotions with no judgmental statements, whether you think she is responding appropriately or not. Remember, there is no right or wrong response for a woman dealing with initial breast cancer diagnosis.

> *My wife told me later that one of the best things I did to help her during those first few days was to cry with her. This seemed to really say to her, 'I'm in this with you. You are not alone.' I knew I had to put her needs first. Listening was important to her. Later I realized this opened the door for good communications for months to come.*
>
> **—AL BARRINEAU**
> **SUPPORT PARTNER**

This is also an extremely hard time for you—particularly the tears, because instinctively your desire is to "make things right" and stop her flow of tears. However, as we have already discussed, tears can be a necessary part of reconciling the loss. Tears are considered a normal, healthy reaction to her diagnosis. Allow her this time and space to experience her emotions in her own way. Some women cry for days or weeks, or every time they talk about their cancer, while others shed few tears, often in private. Whatever her response, let her grieve her loss with you simply staying close by with loving support. Don't ever tell her to stop crying because "it won't help anything." Instead, this response can cause an increase in the emotional pain she is experiencing. Tears are a healthy sign of dealing with a loss for most women.

As women are groping to understand, most support partners report that they are also hurting and do not know exactly what to do or say. Rest assured that everyone searches to understand their new role of support. It is not easy to deal with your own emotions and try to meet the emotional needs of the one you love at the same time. Occasionally, you may be more acutely and visibly distressed than your partner. This is okay. Remember, people respond differently to a frightening crisis. Individuals have their own characteristic ways of coming to grips with an unexpected situation.

WHAT MOST WOMEN WANT

When initially diagnosed, women have said that what they needed most at this emotionally distressing time was not elaborate words or deeds, but reassurance that their loved one would be with them throughout the ordeal. Their greatest need seems to be your silent presence and assurance that you will be with them through this trial. Words don't seem to be as important and are often unheard, but your close presence is remembered and appreciated. Try to give your mate room to grieve in the way she feels necessary without being judgmental. Don't try to tell her what to do unless she asks. Assure her of your continued commitment to the relationship. The magical words are "whatever comes, I am here with you."

ANGER—A POSITIVE SIGN

During the emotionally charged period following diagnosis, your loved one may display angry out-bursts. Loss and fear create anger. Anger needs a target for its expression. This anger may be directed toward herself for not seeking medical attention earlier or for her non-compliance with screening guidelines. It may be directed at her healthcare team for some reason. However, more often her anger may be directed at those closest to her—spouse, children, parents or close friends. This display usually is not meant to be a personal attack but is rather an effort to regain or maintain control.

Often, in her mind, it is not okay to get angry with her doctors, nurses or God. Therefore, that anger may be displaced onto you or family members. View her anger as a positive sign that she is not emotionally succumbing to the diagnosis but is beginning to fight back. Forgive her and don't view the bitterness and frustration as being directed personally toward you. Don't abandon her physically or emotionally if this occurs. This will all pass.

One woman remarked, "In my fit of anger and tears at diagnosis I pushed my husband away emotionally. The one thing that happened that made a difference was a note he left reaffirming his love and the fact that this had made him more aware than ever of how important I was to him, and that he would always be here with me. This allowed me to hear what I was afraid to ask. I needed, more than anything, to be reassured that this would not cause me to lose the most important person in my life; my breast was enough to lose."

Confirmation of your love and continued presence are the best responses you can give your part-ner during the time immediately following diagnosis. Find your own way to convey your message of commitment to her during this crisis—tell her, write her notes, or show her by your actions.

PREDICTING HOW SHE WILL RESPOND

Her emotional response now and during the entire experience will be affected by her personality and prior coping skills. Women respond differently to the diagnosis according to their personalities. Some women may become hysterical and tearful when they hear the words, "You have breast cancer." Others, however, may sit staunchly and show very little emotion in public. Some women want all the available facts, opinions and information they can gather; others want only the basic information needed to make a decision. Too much information can be distressing for some women. Not enough information can be distressing for others.

Some women want their support partner constantly by their side after diagnosis. Others feel a need to withdraw privately to sort through their problems on their own. Some want their partner's verbal input and opinions on treatment options. Others prefer to make their own decisions. Some want their support partner present at every office visit or treatment, and still others feel that this is too emotionally crowding and prefer to go alone unless physically unable.

Some women find it easy to communicate their emotional pain. Others find it difficult to express their feelings. Some find looking at their scar area with their support partner after surgery disturbing and tend to hide to undress. Others feel very comfortable about showing their support partners the scar area and openly dress and undress. There is no right or wrong reaction. Each response originates from complex differences in personalities and is colored by life's experiences.

A woman will also respond to the breast cancer experience based on the value she places on her breast and her body image as well as on how she perceives your response. Age, strangely enough, is not a determining factor of a woman's response to the loss or alteration of a breast. It is a misconception to assume that older women will not be as affected by the impact of surgery as greatly as younger women and are not interested in preserving their body image. This is not true. Some 75 year-old women do not want to have their breast removed and request breast conserving surgery or immediate reconstruction. Personal perception and not age is what determines how women respond.

Some women do not want to leave the hospital after a mastectomy without a temporary prosthesis to camouflage the change in their body image. Oddly enough, some women in their early thirties may request a mastectomy because of their fears of recurrence or radiation therapy, thus placing very little emphasis on body image. They feel comfortable going without a bra after mastectomy. We cannot predict the value a woman places on her body image or her personal perception of the effects of different treatments.

Pressure from you for one procedure or another can add great stress on your partner. As a support partner, it is helpful for you to learn about the options and to be able to discuss them with her. However, it is necessary to allow her to make the final decision and feel she has your support for her decision. When women are allowed to take the lead in the decision of how they want their body images preserved or restored after a diagnosis of breast cancer, they seem to make a better adjustment to the procedure and to their new, altered body images.

The best predictor of how your partner will react throughout the breast cancer experience is how she has responded in the past to life crises. Take this as your clue as to how she will probably respond and the basis for your support plan. If you are unsure about how she will react, what her needs are, or what she expects from you, ask specifically if a certain action will be helpful.

REMEMBER

A WOMAN RESPONDS TO THE DIAGNOSIS OF BREAST CANCER ACCORDING TO HER BASIC PERSONALITY AND PREVIOUS COPING EXPERIENCES.

HER RESPONSE IS GREATLY INFLUENCED HOW HER PERCEPTION OF HOW BREAST SURGERY WILL CHANGE HER PERSONAL BODY IMAGE AND HOW SHE FEELS YOU WILL RESPOND TO THE CHANGE.

THERE IS NO RIGHT OR WRONG WAY TO RESPOND EMOTIONALLY TO A DIAGNOSIS.

AS A SUPPORT PARTNER, YOU NEED TO CREATE A "SAFE SPACE" FOR HER TO WORK THROUGH HER EMOTIONS.

MOST WOMEN DESIRE YOUR SILENT, CARING PRESENCE MORE THAN ELABORATE WORDS OR DEEDS.

ANGRY OUTBURSTS ARE A SIGN THAT SHE IS FIGHTING BACK RATHER THAN SUCCUMBING TO THE DIAGNOSIS.

CONFIRMATION OF YOUR LOVE AND CONTINUED SUPPORT IS VITAL, WHATEVER HER RESPONSE.

WEALTH
KNOWLEDGE
COMPETENCE

ARE ALL SUBSERVIENT

TO THE QUALITY OF

FAITHFUL SUPPORT

WHEN A PERSON

IS IN NEED.

WE ARE NOT PRIMARILY

PUT HERE ON EARTH

TO SEE THROUGH

ONE ANOTHER,

BUT RATHER TO SEE

ONE ANOTHER THROUGH.

— AUTHOR UNKNOWN

WHAT DO I DO FIRST?

What do you need to do first? One support partner said, "When I heard the words 'breast cancer' from the physician, I felt I had to do everything to protect the one I loved from the hurt. I became mobilized for action. I had to do something. I became very verbal in my opinions as to what she needed to do next, on the way home from the physician. The problem came when I took actions, which later I found were not needed or appropriate for her diagnosis. I learned I had added much pressure to the pain she was feeling."

As a support partner, you may feel compelled to act to make things better. However, in order to take the appropriate steps, you must allow her time to come to grips with the emotional impact, as we just discussed. Assess what you can do that will be most helpful to her. The question, "How can I be most helpful to you at this time?" may prevent many problems by offering the kind of support she really wants and needs.

> *Despite all the macho training our society provides, there are some things we can't fix. My persistent urge was to make it all right, but I was forced to learn that cancer was one of those things I could not 'fix.'*
>
> **—BRIAN CLUXTON**
> **SUPPORT PARTNER**

The patient has had no preparation to deal with all of the emotions and complex decision-making demands that accompany the diagnosis. Therefore, as the primary support person, you may be most helpful by locating sources of information specific to her diagnosis. The best source for accurate information is the treatment team. Identify someone on the treatment team with whom you can comfortably communicate and who can recommend additional resources.

The overwhelming desire to "make things better" needs to be directed with correct information. Take time to learn the basics of the disease, treatment options, and what steps need to be taken in what time frame. Very seldom is breast cancer a medical emergency (an exception is

REMEMBER

ALLOW HER TIME TO
ABSORB THE
EMOTIONAL IMPACT.
SHE NEEDS TIME TO CRY
AND EXPRESS HER
FEELINGS.

OBTAIN CORRECT
INFORMATION FROM YOUR
TREATMENT TEAM
BEFORE SURGING AHEAD
WITH ADVICE OR
DECISION-MAKING.

ASSESS HOW YOU
CAN BEST HELP.
RESIST THE URGE TO RUSH
THE PATIENT OR TO
INSIST ON ANY
PARTICULAR TREATMENT
OPTION.

inflammatory breast cancer, which requires immediate treatment). Most women have time to learn about their disease and consider various treatment options before submitting to surgery, chemotherapy, or radiation treatments.

In most cases, breast cancer has been in a woman's body for years. A tumor that has a normal growing cycle (doubles every 100 days) and is one centimeter in size (3/8 inch, the size of the tip of a woman's smallest finger) could have been in her body for eight or more years and has just now become detectable. Several more weeks in which to gather information and make educated, appropriate decisions will not adversely affect the outcome for the patient. Women who receive support while reviewing their options, without pressure on specifics from their support partner, will have the foundation needed for emotional recovery.

> *My wife has always coped extremely well during times of crisis. She becomes very organized. She develops a plan of action and puts it into motion. She immediately seeks as much information as she can regarding the crisis. I knew this was one of the first things she needed from me—my help and support as we tried to find out about this enemy that had invaded her body.*
>
> **—AL BARRINEAU**
> **SUPPORT PARTNER**

DEALING WITH
THE CHILDREN

For partners with children the most common question is, "What do we tell the children?" The truth! Children are very perceptive. They know and sense much more than they could ever communicate. They will immediately feel that something is wrong in the family even if you decide not to tell them. What they imagine may be much worse than the truth. From the beginning, it is imperative that you be open and honest with them about what is occurring in the family.

They need to hear the truth from you or your partner on a language level they can understand. You do not have to tell everything that is happening, but you need to give them enough information so they will feel a part of the family. Finding out from someone outside the family can weaken a child's trust, resulting in a lowered trust factor in the future.

TIPS FOR TELLING THE CHILDREN:

- If possible, wait until you and your mate have some control of your emotions. For some, this may take a day or two; others may be able to share the first day.

- Ask your treatment team for information, or call your local American Cancer Society for information written for children about a parent's cancer.

- With your mate, plan what you will say to the children. Plan a time when both of you can share with them and not be interrupted.

- Turn off the television and take the telephone off the hook to prevent interruptions.

- Start by sharing something similar to the following: "Mommie has found a lump in her breast. The doctor says that the lump is cancer (call it by the right name). Cancer cells grow too fast. The doctors say that they need to take this lump out because these are not good cells. The doctors and nurses can also help by giving medicine." Continue to share truthfully and simply what the facts are. If you have an example that will help explain, this will be helpful.

- If you or your mate begins to cry, assure your children that this is because you are sad and it is okay to be sad and to cry.

- Allow the children to ask questions. Answer to the best of your ability. If you do not know the answers, be honest and say you do not know.

- Reassure them that you will continue to tell them what is happening.

- Involve them in the process of helping Mom adjust to surgery and possible treatments. Help them to feel as if they are part of the solution to the problem by sharing chores that contribute to the well-being of the family.

> *Being open and honest with our children helped us all. My wife had always been there for us. Now it was time for us to be her support and strength. Taking care of Mom helped the boys to deal with their emotions.*
>
> **—AL BARRINEAU**
> **SUPPORT PARTNER**

Teenage children and grown children also need to communicate openly and honestly. However, don't be surprised if they don't seem to be overly concerned and quickly return to their normal duties and interests. Take this as a compliment; your openness has restored their confidence that, as a family, you can cope with your new situation.

It is suggested that you inform the teachers or instructors of your children that your child is dealing with a cancer diagnosis (or family crisis) at home. This alerts them and allows them to identify potential changes in a child's behavior as a stress reaction to the change in their home environments. This knowledge allows them to offer support and understanding if a child should act out, rather than correction. They will also be able to recognize if the child is suffering from overwhelming sadness and needs emotional support. Older children and teens may feel more comfortable sharing their feelings with adults outside the home rather than with their parents. This information allows this person to offer valuable emotional support to your child.

Teachers are also often in a position to request help and assistance from other school personnel, such as trained professional counselors and school psychologists, in order to offer additional professional emotional support to a child.

IMPACT OF DIAGNOSIS ON CHILDREN

Families often worry about the effect the illness will have on their children. The most important factor in how they respond is how they see you and your partner respond to the illness. If they see you communicating openly, honestly, and sharing with a positive attitude, they will be more likely to respond the same way. The family can value this time as one of growth and maturity in problem solving. If you find it difficult to know what to say or realize problems are developing in the family with the children, contact your cancer treatment center and ask for a counselor trained in dealing with children.

In his book, *How Do We Tell The Children?*, David Pertz, M.D., explains:

> *"A child's first question about illness and death is an attempt to gain mastery over frightening images of abandonment, separation, loneliness, pain and bodily damage. If we err on the side of overprotecting them from emotional pain and grief with 'kind lies' we risk weakening their coping capacities."*

SUPPORT FOR CHILDREN:

Kids Konnected

27071 Cabot Road # 102
Laguna Hills, CA 92653

800-899-2866 - Fax: 949-582-3989
www.kidskonnected.org

Offers: Free Teddy Bears 3 - 18 yrs.
Internet Web Site
Books - Hot Line - Newsletters
Summer Camps - Grief Workshops
Leadership Training

REMEMBER

CHILDREN NEED TO BE TOLD THE TRUTH BY YOU OR YOUR PARTNER.

AN ILLNESS NEED NOT ADVERSELY AFFECT CHILDREN.

CHILDREN USUALLY RESPOND IN A MANNER SIMILAR TO THE WAY THEY OBSERVE THE PARENTS RESPONDING.

INFORM TEACHERS AND INSTRUCTORS OF THE DIAGNOSIS SO THEY CAN OFFER ADDITIONAL UNDERSTANDING AND SUPPORT.

A CRISIS CAN SERVE AS A TIME OF GROWTH AND EMOTIONAL MATURITY IN A FAMILY UNIT.

SUPPORT PARTNERS

BUILD BRIDGES OF HOPE

AND REASSURANCE

WHEN OTHERS

ARE VULNERABLE,

EXPOSED AND

SELF-CONSCIOUS.

SUPPORT PARTNERS

TAKE AN INTEREST IN YOU, BUT

NOT A CONTROLLING INTEREST.

— JUDY KNEECE

DEALING WITH HEALTH INSURANCE AND EMPLOYMENT

As you are dealing with the emotionally overwhelming issues of breast cancer treatment, you may find it equally overwhelming to cope with the financial changes incurred by a diagnosis of cancer. Most patients have some form of health insurance coverage to help with the medical expenses. Bills will come from the hospital, physicians, pharmacies, treatment centers, etc. Your challenge is keeping accurate records to ensure optimal reimbursement of claims. This often means constant communication between your insurance carrier and those billing you for services. As a support partner, you can play a vital role by organizing the record keeping, thereby reducing the stress brought on your partner by the barrage of bills and claims.

If you are insured at the time of diagnosis, call your insurance provider or carefully read your policy for guidelines. You need the following information:

● Requirements and procedure for pre-approval for hospital admissions

● Requirements for second opinions for surgery or treatments

● Guidelines for second opinions from physicians

> *Being properly insured relieved us of one of the biggest problems a lot of people face–the financial responsibility of dealing with a serious illness. We were fortunate. But even if we had no insurance coverage, I would not have let that keep us from getting the medical attention my wife needed. Outstanding bills would have been a small price to pay for her life.*
>
> **—AL BARRINEAU**
> **SUPPORT PARTNER**

- Procedure for filing claims

- Claim forms to be mailed to you

- Name of person at the insurance company who will handle your claims

- Amount of deductibles, if any, before claims are paid

- Limits imposed on amounts paid for surgery, chemotherapy, radiation therapy, or reconstructive surgery

- Coverage for new or "experimental treatments" or for clinical trials. Ask what they cover and if there are any limits on amounts for such procedures

RECORD KEEPING

Keeping up with the filing of claims and payments can become burdensome. However, accurate record-keeping and careful scrutiny of all bills makes the task much simpler. The following suggestions may be helpful:

- Purchase a pocket calendar to be used to record all appointments (decide if you or the patient will keep the calendar).

- Write on the calendar: physician visits, procedures performed, medications administered, or supplies used.

- Provide your physicians with appropriate claim forms and ask if they will file them for you.

- At the time of service, ask for a copy of all charges, or ask to have one mailed to you.

- Keep copies of all charges for appointments, services, medications or medical supplies in one place (a designated box, file folder, or drawer will serve this purpose).

- Check periodically to see if appropriate payments are being made to medical providers.

- If problems arise with payments, contact your healthcare facility or provider and ask for help in providing the information needed to receive adequate payment.

- Call your insurance provider and talk with your claims representative to offer additional records or assistance for getting information from your medical providers. (Always record the name of the person to whom you speak. You may need the name for future reference.)

- Keep all premiums current. Do not allow your insurance to lapse from lack of payment.

- Insurance coverage is more difficult to obtain after any major illness. For this reason be very careful to keep all premiums current. Before your partner or you as the primary policyholder decide to change jobs, be sure she will be covered under the new employer's insurance program. If you decide to leave your present employer, ask about continuing your present policy until the new one becomes effective. Some policies may not cover a pre-existing condition or illness.

FINANCIAL NEEDS

If you realize that this is going to be a financial burden to your family, or if you are uninsured, ask to speak to the social worker in the cancer treatment center as soon as possible. Social workers are trained to help with the social issues of the illness, including helping to secure financial help for medical services if needed. There are various services available for cancer patients. The earlier you can make this need known, the more effective the social work team can be in helping you. Application for help often requires filing forms and a period of waiting for approval. People often feel embarrassed to ask for help and postpone the issue. However, many people find that an unexpected illness drains their financial reserves. You are not alone. Ask for help early.

> *When it came to the bills that come with a cancer diagnosis my attitude was 'who cares' Get the needed treatment, no matter what, and we will worry about the bills when they arrive. Anna needed to know that no price was too great to pay for her future health.*
>
> **—BRIAN CLUXTON**
> **SUPPORT PARTNER**

EMPLOYMENT ISSUES

A woman in treatment for breast cancer will be away from her job for some period of time, which varies among patients. Surgery can result in an absence of three to six weeks according to the type of surgery, healing time, and the nature of her employment. Her surgeon will estimate when she will be able to return to work. Her supervisor needs to be informed of the expected sick leave time that will be necessary following surgery and/or treatment. If treatment is required after surgery, additional time may be needed since chemotherapy and radiation side effects vary in patients. The oncologist will need to be consulted as to how much time away from work can be expected. Some women are able to work a normal schedule during treatments. Others have to curtail their activities because of treatment, taking sick leave for the treatment period. A woman's physical and emotional demands at work, plus the type of drugs in her treatment plan, and her general health will determine if she can continue to work. Only her doctors can provide anticipated time needed for recovery.

REMEMBER

WISE PLANNING AND RECORD KEEPING
CAN REMOVE MOST OF THE HASSLE
FROM INSURANCE REIMBURSEMENTS.

SUPPORT PARTNERS CAN TAKE MUCH
STRESS OFF THE PATIENT BY PERFORMING
RECORD-KEEPING TASKS.

KEEP ALL INSURANCE
PREMIUMS CURRENT.

IF YOU NEED FINANCIAL HELP,
ASK A SOCIAL WORKER
AT YOUR CANCER TREATMENT CENTER
AS EARLY AS POSSIBLE.

TIME AWAY FROM WORK VARIES
WITH DIFFERENT TYPES OF TREATMENT.
PHYSICIANS CAN HELP
PREDICT TIME NEEDED FOR SICK LEAVE.

ISSUES OF DISCRIMINATION
IN EMPLOYMENT CAN BE
BROUGHT TO THE ATTENTION
OF PROFESSIONALS IN THE AREA
OF PROTECTION FOR CANCER PATIENTS.

ASK YOUR PARTNER HOW MUCH
INFORMATION SHE WOULD LIKE FOR HER
FRIENDS OR CO-WORKERS TO KNOW
ABOUT HER ILLNESS.

WORKPLACE DISCRIMINATION

Occasionally, a cancer patient may be discriminated against at her workplace because of illness. However, there are both federal and state laws to protect her. The social worker at the cancer treatment center will be able to help you in this matter. In addition, there are names and telephone numbers of national organizations that deal with these issues listed in the reference section of this book.

TELLING FELLOW EMPLOYEES AND FRIENDS

Ask your partner what she wants her co-workers and concerned friends to know about her diagnosis and treatment. Some women are very open with their co-workers and friends and talk freely about their disease and its treatment. Other women feel that this is private and prefer to keep the details to themselves. Knowing her wishes is helpful because friends and co-workers will come to visit and call to ask about the patient. Being aware of what she wants others to know allows you to answer their questions without invading her privacy. Some women feel it helpful if their support partner communicates with the office during their illnesses, especially during the acute diagnostic period. Patients soon tire of "telling their illness story" and find it a relief to have someone perform this role.

SUPPORT GROUPS

For some, it may be hard to reach out to others during the breast cancer experience. Often, you doubt if a support group would be very beneficial to you. You may feel you have enough support, or cannot relate to a support group. However, many find that a support group is one of the most effective methods for emotional management.

Support groups that are disease specific, such as one for breast cancer patients, are composed of people who are going through the same problems of learning to live life under similar circumstances. You and your partner may benefit from a support group. Studies have proven that participating in support groups improves the quality of life and relationships of patients. "Sometimes fear is so engulfing it precludes the ability to call for help," explains one patient. "It is this fear that those of us called patients understand and can help to diminish for one another" (Robert Fisher, Patient To Patient Volunteer Program).

Support groups are a place where people with similar fears and needs meet and share to reduce their anguish and confusion. They are places where all anxieties, anger, and apprehensiveness are understood without any raised eyebrows as to their significance, and a place to increase your knowledge and perception of the disease that she is battling. Families and friends are wonderful sources of support, but only someone going through the same life crisis can fully comprehend and empathize. That's the role of support groups. Finding a group for your partner and one for yourself will add a new dimension to your breast cancer experience.

> *Getting involved in a support group for mates of breast cancer patients provided a haven for me. I had felt a need to be the strong one for my wife. The support group gave me the opportunity and place to express my concerns, ask my questions, and voice my fears. I was with others who could truly relate to the way I felt: people who really understood.*
>
> **—AL BARRINEAU**
> **SUPPORT PARTNER**

REMEMBER

FOR MANY, SUPPORT
GROUPS OFFER A SAFE
PLACE TO EXPRESS
FEELINGS AND RECEIVE
SUPPORT.

LOOK FOR A SUPPORT
GROUP THAT HAS AN
EDUCATIONAL COMPONENT
AS PART OF THE MEETING.

Look for a support group that is led by a professional facilitator who is trained in group dynamics and who knows how to keep the meeting meaningful to those present. A group should offer an opportunity to share experiences, but should not be dominated by "poor me" stories. Instead, educational and support techniques should be provided at each meeting. You may want to talk with the facilitator before attending a meeting to determine if the characteristics of the particular group meet your needs.

For information on breast cancer support groups, contact your cancer treatment center, the local American Cancer Society, or the National Alliance of Breast Cancer Organizations. (Addresses and phone numbers are listed in the reference section of this book along with other support and educational resources.)

UNDERSTANDING BREAST CANCER

Breast cancer is a very complex disease with many variables involved in its treatment. The language and terminology used by the medical profession is often unique to the disease. This chapter is designed to clarify and explain the basic facts of breast cancer in the simplest way.

Cancer begins when normal cells in the breast change into cells that have an uncontrolled growth pattern. The cancer cells continue to divide and grow and may spread to other parts of the breast and then to other parts of the body if not removed. The cancer cells can invade neighboring tissues and spread throughout the body, establishing new growths at distant sites, a process called metastasis.

BREAST CANCER

Most people think that all breast cancers are the same. However, there are approximately 15 different identified types of breast cancer. Cancers that develop from different types of breast tissue in different parts of the breast may have varying characteristics. The term carcinoma is used by physicians to describe a malignant or cancerous growth.

> *Somehow I thought that if I learned enough about breast cancer and all its treatments, we could beat it with knowledge. I was on a mission, I read tons of books and surfed the Internet, looking for the magical answer. However, I soon found that the Internet could be a very scary place for support partners of the newly diagnosed. There is a lot of misinformation out there, so stick to recommended sources of help.*
>
> —BRIAN CLUXTON
> SUPPORT PARTNER

NORMAL BREAST ANATOMY

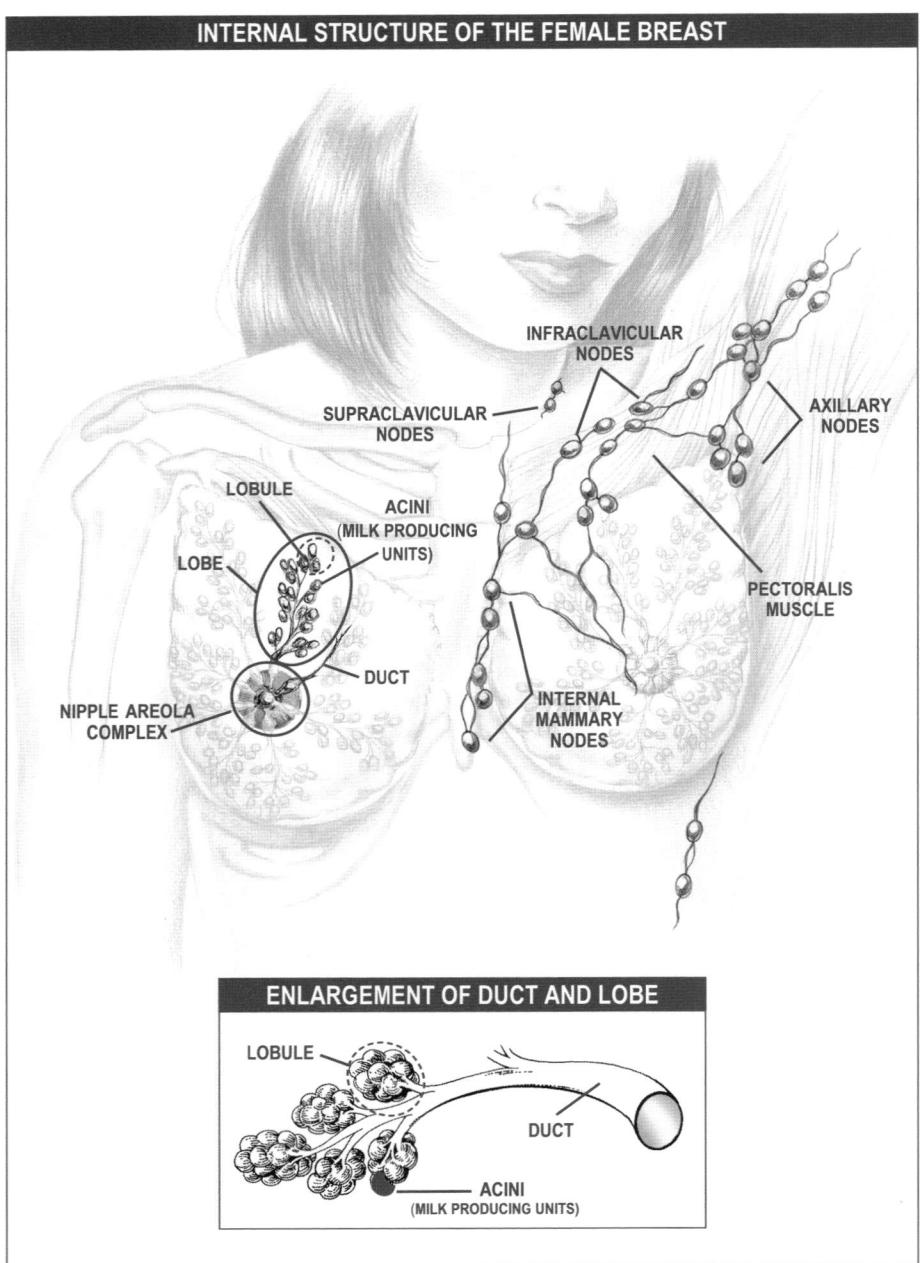

INTERNAL STRUCTURE OF THE FEMALE BREAST

INFRACLAVICULAR NODES

SUPRACLAVICULAR NODES

AXILLARY NODES

LOBULE

ACINI (MILK PRODUCING UNITS)

LOBE

DUCT

NIPPLE AREOLA COMPLEX

PECTORALIS MUSCLE

INTERNAL MAMMARY NODES

ENLARGEMENT OF DUCT AND LOBE

LOBULE

DUCT

ACINI (MILK PRODUCING UNITS)

TYPES OF CANCERS:

Cancers are first classified according to their relationship to walls of their origin. The two major divisions are: in situ and invasive/infiltrating.

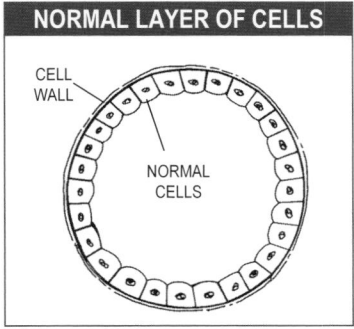

NORMAL LAYER OF CELLS

CELL WALL

NORMAL CELLS

Normal ducts and lobules are lined with one or more layers of orderly cells.

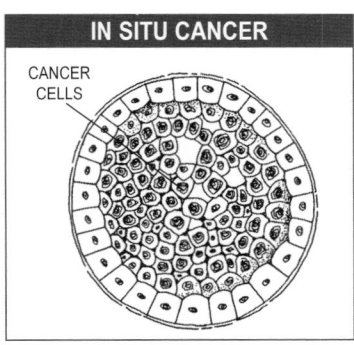

IN SITU CANCER

CANCER CELLS

In situ carcinomas are cancers that are still contained within the walls of the portion of the breast in which they developed. The cancer has not grown through the cell wall and invaded surrounding tissue.

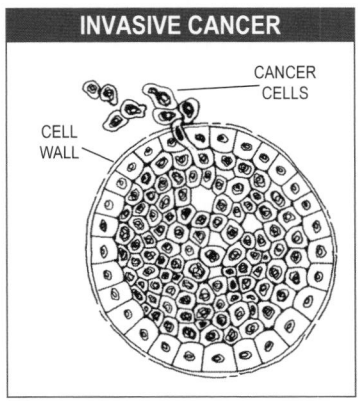

INVASIVE CANCER

CANCER CELLS

CELL WALL

Infiltrating or invasive carcinomas are cancers that have grown through the duct or lobular walls and into surrounding tissues.

DESCRIPTIONS OF CANCERS:

Breast cancers are named according to the part of the breast in which they develop.

DUCTAL CARCINOMA	LOBULAR CARCINOMA

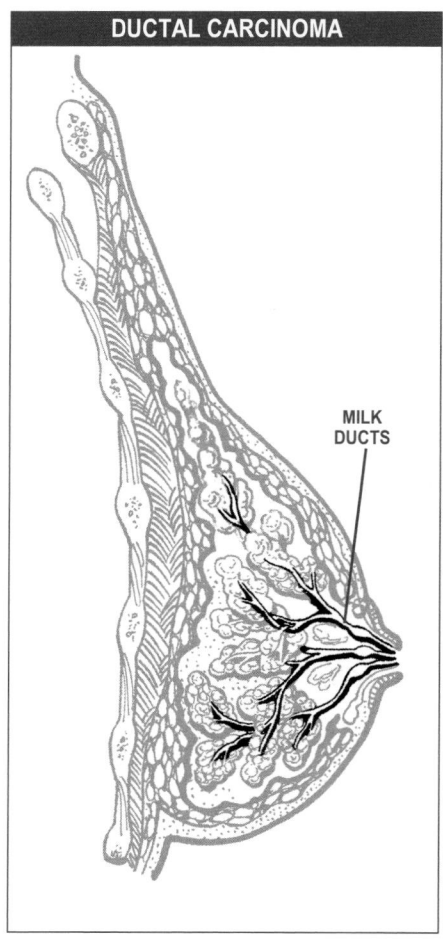

MILK
DUCTS

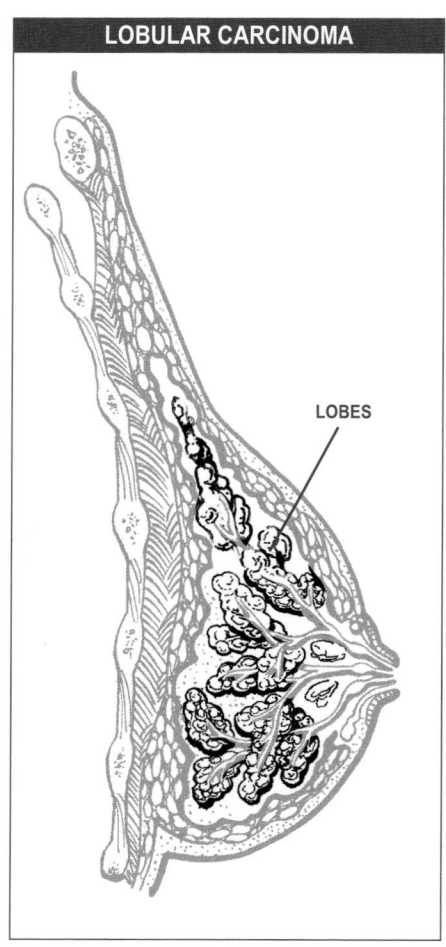

LOBES

Ductal carcinomas begin in the ducts of the breast and comprise the majority of breast cancers.

Lobular carcinomas begin in the lobules of the breast and occur a small percentage of the time.

INVASIVE AND IN SITU CANCERS

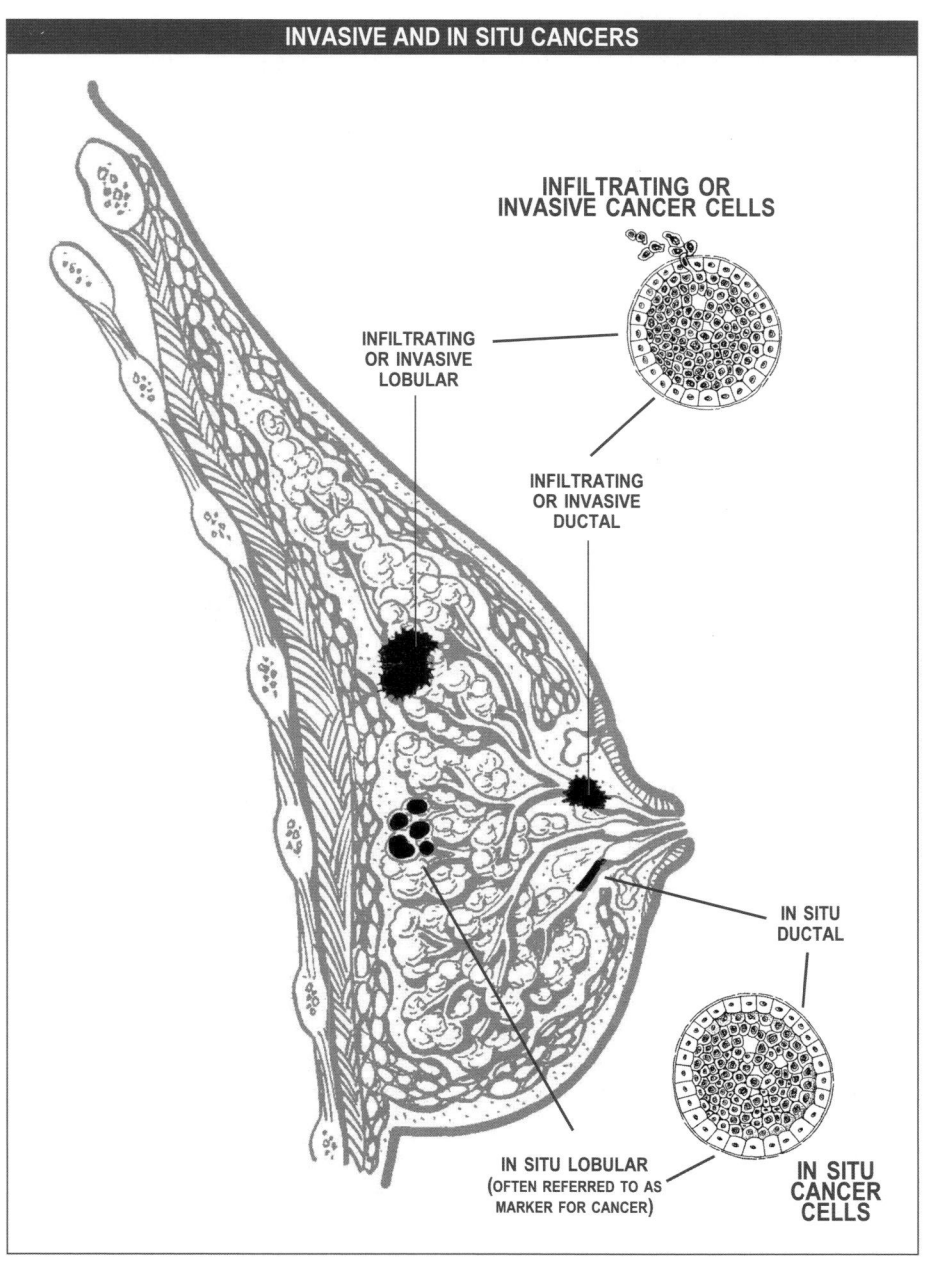

INFILTRATING OR
INVASIVE CANCER CELLS

INFILTRATING
OR INVASIVE
LOBULAR

INFILTRATING
OR INVASIVE
DUCTAL

IN SITU
DUCTAL

IN SITU LOBULAR
(OFTEN REFERRED TO AS
MARKER FOR CANCER)

IN SITU
CANCER
CELLS

GROWTH OF BREAST CANCER

Some breast cancers grow rapidly, while others grow very slowly. Breast cancers have been shown to double in size every 23 to 209 days. A tumor that doubles every 100 days (the estimated average doubling time) has been in a woman's body approximately eight to ten years when it reaches one centimeter in size (3/8 inch), which is the size of the tip of her smallest finger. The cancer begins with one damaged cell and doubles until it is detected on mammography, by finding a lump, or from symptoms such as a discharge or a change in the breast.

Some believe that cancers may grow in spurts and the doubling time may vary at different times. However, when a one centimeter tumor is found, the tumor has already grown from one cell to approximately 100 billion cells.

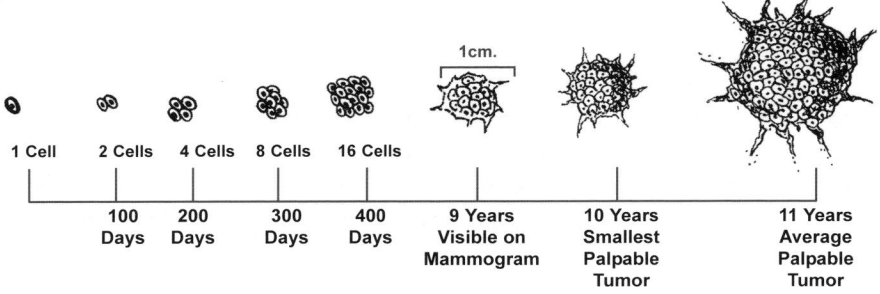

1 Cell	2 Cells	4 Cells	8 Cells	16 Cells			
	100 Days	200 Days	300 Days	400 Days	9 Years Visible on Mammogram	10 Years Smallest Palpable Tumor	11 Years Average Palpable Tumor

Breast cancer is not a sudden occurrence, but is a process that has been developing for a period of time. Therefore, when a biopsy confirms a cancerous breast tumor, your mate is most often not facing a medical emergency. You have time to get answers to your questions and learn about the particular disease and treatment options. Most physicians recommend surgery within several weeks of the biopsy. There are exceptions, such as inflammatory carcinoma (cancer in the lymphatic system), which requires immediate treatment with chemotherapy for maximum control. Ask the physician what recommendations will be made regarding your partner's particular tumor. Tests performed on the tumor will reveal cell type and estimate whether the tumor is a very slow growing or a more rapidly growing tumor.

"We were shocked and over-whelmed by what we needed to know and what we didn't know about breast cancer.

—AL BARRINEAU
SUPPORT PARTNER

Some tumors will have the characteristic of spreading quickly to other parts of the body. Others do not seem to spread as readily. Breast cancer spreads to other parts of the body through the lymphatic system or the blood system. The spread of the cancer can be local (in the area of the breast), regional (in the nodes or area near the breast), or distant (to other organs of the body). These characteristics will be presented in the pathology report after surgery.

After a biopsy confirming cancer, a woman will usually have to make some decisions about treatment options. These decisions will include surgical procedures, and possibly radiation therapy, chemotherapy, or hormonal therapy. Surgical decisions will be based on the preliminary (biopsy) study of the tumor.

When the final (surgical) pathology report is evaluated, the oncologist will decide which treatments are most appropriate for your partner's type of cancer. For some cancers, surgery may be the only treatment needed. Others may require additional treatment with radiation therapy, chemotherapy, or hormonal therapy.

REMEMBER

BREAST CANCER IS USUALLY NOT A MEDICAL EMERGENCY. YOU HAVE TIME TO GET THE ANSWERS TO YOUR QUESTIONS BEFORE FINAL TREATMENT IS SELECTED.

THE BIOPSY PATHOLOGY REPORT IS USED TO MAKE SURGICAL DECISIONS.

THE FINAL PATHOLOGY REPORT IS USED TO DETERMINE TREATMENT WITH CHEMOTHERAPY, RADIATION, OR HORMONAL DECISIONS.

SUPPORT PARTNERS

TWO ARE BETTER THAN ONE,
BECAUSE THEY GET A
GOOD RETURN FOR THEIR WORK:

IF ONE FALLS DOWN,
HIS FRIEND CAN HELP HIM UP.

BUT PITY THE MAN
WHO FALLS AND HAS
NO ONE TO HELP HIM UP!

ALSO,
IF TWO LIE DOWN TOGETHER,
THEY WILL KEEP WARM.
BUT HOW CAN ONE
KEEP WARM ALONE?

THOUGH ONE
MAY BE OVERPOWERED,
TWO CAN DEFEND THEMSELVES.

A CORD OF THREE STRANDS
IS NOT QUICKLY BROKEN.

— ECCLESIASTES 4: 9-12

BREAST CANCER DECISIONS

Many women reveal that after they heard their physician say the word "cancer," they remember very little about what was discussed during the remainder of the visit. However, it is essential that information about the extent of the disease and treatment options that is provided in this first meeting be accurately understood. Treatment decisions and necessary steps of actions are dependent on a complete understanding of what was said by your partner's physician. If you were present when the physician discussed your partner's diagnosis, you can help remember the information relayed. Discuss with your partner what the physician said so you can be assured that you both have the same understanding of the decisions that need to be made shortly.

However, if you feel that you were also overwhelmed and do not have a reliable recall, clarification of information from the physician is necessary. Call your physician to schedule a return visit; it is vital to have this information before treatment options can be explored. Sometimes a period of time, usually overnight, may need to pass in order for questions to surface that need to be answered. Often the physician's nurse will be able to answer many of your questions.

If a return call or visit is necessary, be prepared to ask all of the questions that have emerged during your discussions. Take notes or tape-record (ask permission) the answers. You may want to continue the practice of note taking or recording your consultations with the physician or nurse. In addition, ask for written information on breast

> *The best thing our doctors did to help us in the beginning was to keep our primary physician informed. He was the one I looked to, the one I relied on. Their cooperation and good communication were invaluable during our decision-making processes.*
>
> —AL BARRINEAU
> SUPPORT PARTNER

55

cancer, options for surgery, and treatment recommendations following surgery. Becoming informed partners with your healthcare team is essential in order to regain a sense of control.

Most women eagerly seek help from their partners in gathering information. Some, however, do not want any assistance past the information gathering stage. They prefer to make treatment decisions completely on their own. Therefore, communication about the desired level of participation between the two of you is crucial if the support is to be helpful to the patient.

THE DECISION-MAKING PROCESS

There will be many decisions and conversations with your healthcare team. Therefore, it will be helpful if you begin to read and acquire a basic understanding of the terminology and types of treatments. Your partner's anxiety level may be so high that she cannot participate in the search for information nor comprehend what she reads or hears. Included at the back of this book is a glossary of basic terms used in the diagnosis and treatment of breast cancer. It will be helpful to familiarize yourself with these terms.

It is very important that the information you collect is specific to her diagnosis. There are approximately 15 types of breast cancer. Furthermore, treatments can vary even with the same type of cancer. Many factors are considered when developing a treatment plan. Ask your partner's physician for the specifics of the diagnosis. Remember, her healthcare team should always be your primary source of information. There are some important questions regarding the specifics of her initial diagnosis that are helpful to know.

QUESTIONS TO ASK YOUR HEALTHCARE TEAM ABOUT IMMEDIATE DECISIONS

- What is the name of her cancer?
- Do you have written information on her cancer?
- Is the cancer in situ (inside of the cell walls) or invasive (grown through the cell walls)?
- What is the size of the tumor?
- Is there any suspected lymph node involvement?
- Is cancer suspected in any other area of the same breast or the opposite breast?
- Is there evidence that the cancer has spread outside the breast and nodes?
- Where can we get written information on her cancer type and treatment options?
- What decisions will she need to make about her upcoming treatment? (Surgery is usually the first decision. Lumpectomy versus mastectomy; if mastectomy, reconstruction immediate or delayed. Other decisions are made after final pathology report is available).

- In what time frame do you recommend that the decisions be made?
- Who on the healthcare team can answer our questions?
- When and how can he/she be contacted for questions or information? (Telephone, personal appointments, e-mail, etc.).
- Are there any characteristics about her cancer that could impact our decision-making that we should be aware of?
- Will her case be presented to a multidisciplinary conference for evaluation by a team of physicians? (Breast centers usually have conferences before surgery and treatment where a team of physicians from all disciplines review her case as a group and offer suggestions to her physicians for treatment options. This conference is usually without charge and is offered as a service to the patient.)
- If she desires a second opinion, how and what should be done to arrange one?
- Do you have recommended books to read about these decisions?

This information will be combined with the age, menopausal status, general health, and treatment goals of the patient to help determine treatment recommendations. Before anyone can give you accurate information on suggested treatment, these basic facts need to be known. Without access to the mammography film and/or report and a final biopsy pathology report describing all aspects of the tumor, any information about her particular case can only be an educated guess.

The media—including television, radio and magazines—has taken up the cause of breast cancer education. However, much of this information is very general and may not apply to your partner's diagnosis. The information may include non-approved treatments or discoveries unavailable for public use.

Also, be careful of well-meaning friends and their advice. Unless they are professionals in the field of breast cancer, they may offer information that is not applicable and may only confuse you. Remember, the healthcare team is your best source for accurate advice based on your partner's specific diagnosis and her health status. Don't hesitate to get the information you need to make decisions.

If you need more information or clarification on any of the information you read, call the physician's office, cancer treatment center, or organizations specializing in cancer. Sources for free information are available from various professional organizations. Listed in the back of this book are names and addresses of these organizations. One of the most helpful booklets is *Breast Cancer: Treatment Guidelines for Patients,* produced by the American Cancer Society and published in partnership with the National Comprehensive Cancer Network (NCCN). It provides patients and the general public with up-to-date treatment information on breast cancer in understandable terms. Call your local American Cancer Society at 1-800-ACS-2345 for a free copy of NCCN Breast Cancer Treatment Guidelines or download a copy from one of the following Web sites: www.cancer.org or www.nccn.org. The information is a consensus of recommended treatments from 19 comprehensive cancer treatment centers. These guidelines should only serve as a resource for understanding optional treatments for each stage of breast cancer. Each patient must be individually evaluated. Discuss the guidelines or other information with her physician.

SECOND OPINIONS

The question of whether or not a second opinion is needed usually comes up. When a medical diagnosis is serious and the suggested therapy difficult to accept, second opinions can serve a valuable role. Surgery, chemotherapy, and radiation therapy deserve serious consideration. Accurate and specific information will give her confidence that she is making the best and most informed decisions.

A second opinion is obtained from another physician who practices medicine in the same field. After reviewing all her records, treatment advice will be given by this physician. The second opinion can give her reassurance about her treatment decisions. However, for some people, a second opinion may cause anxiety and increase confusion. Some insurance providers require a second opinion before treatment. Check with your insurance company. Physicians may also refer patients for a second opinion to validate treatment decisions. You and your partner should evaluate your needs to determine whether a second opinion will be helpful in your decision-making process.

> *Anna had wonderful doctors she trusted, but we still felt safer having a second opinion. It helped her feel safe proceeding with recommended treatments. We shop for cars, so why not feel comfortable shopping for the best doctors and treatment options?*
>
> —BRIAN CLUXTON
> SUPPORT PARTNER

REASONS FOR A SECOND OPINION MAY INCLUDE:

- Your mate feels insecure or unsure about what she has been told about treatment options
- Your insurance provider requires a second opinion before treatment
- There have been questions or a disagreement within your treatment team about the recommended options for your treatment
- Your mate wants to learn more about newer therapies not offered by your treatment team

If your mate feels a second opinion would resolve her indecisiveness, ask your treatment team for the name of several physicians qualified in this area. You may also call a major cancer treatment center for a referral. Comprehensive breast centers have pretreatment multidisciplinary conferences where a group of physicians from various specialties in breast cancer examine the records, discuss the case and make treatment recommendations after a biopsy and before surgery.

The most common benefit of a second opinion is to have peace of mind in knowing that all needed information was obtained before a decision was made. An informed decision allows patients to go through treatments confident that they chose the best treatment option for themselves. If you sense that there are lingering questions or concerns about decisions, encourage, but don't force, your mate to seek a second opinion. These questions or concerns, if not answered to her satisfaction, will often be a source of emotional discomfort in later months. It is helpful to take the time and effort to get answers to her questions now rather than to rush into treatment decisions with a sense of doubt.

Some women feel comfortable with the initial treatment recommendations, believe their questions have been answered sufficiently, and have no need for a second opinion. This is perfectly acceptable. Seeking a second opinion is an individual decision and one that the patient needs to make according to her needs.

REMEMBER

REQUEST WRITTEN INFORMATION FROM YOUR HEALTHCARE TEAM.

OBTAIN A COPY OF *BREAST CANCER: TREATMENT GUIDELINES FOR PATIENTS* FROM THE AMERICAN CANCER SOCIETY OR THE NATIONAL COMPREHENSIVE CANCER NETWORK.

TAKE TIME TO FAMILIARIZE YOURSELF WITH THE TERMINOLOGY OF BREAST CANCER.

SECOND OPINIONS MAY OR MAY NOT BE HELPFUL IN THE DECISION-MAKING PROCESS.

YOU MUST HAVE ACCURATE INFORMATION UPON WHICH TO MAKE DECISIONS. ONLY YOUR PHYSICIAN AND HEALTHCARE TEAM CAN PROVIDE YOU WITH THE SPECIFICS OF YOUR MATE'S DIAGNOSIS.

COMMUNICATE OPENLY WITH YOUR PARTNER ABOUT THE EXTENT OF YOUR INVOLVEMENT DURING THE DECISION-MAKING PROCESS.

THE ART OF COMMUNICATING

IS NOT ONLY

SAYING THE RIGHT THING

AT THE RIGHT TIME,

BUT ALSO,

LEAVING UNSAID

THE WRONG THING

AT A TEMPTING MOMENT.

— JUDY KNEECE

SURGICAL DECISIONS

Usually, the first decision for the treatment of breast cancer will be the type of surgical procedure to pursue. Breast surgery is the most effective method for treatment of breast cancer. Breast conserving surgery, commonly referred to as a lumpectomy or breast conservation, removes the lump and an area of surrounding tissue (margins). A mastectomy removes the entire breast.

Surgical decisions are dependent on many factors:

- **Type of tumor**—The type is diagnosed by biopsy and confirmed by the final surgical pathology report. There are approximately 15 cell types of breast cancer that vary in characteristics of tumor growth rate and tumor aggressiveness (how likely the tumor may spread to other organs and its potential for occurring in the other breast).

- **Size of the tumor**—Sizes are given in centimeters and millimeters. (Ten millimeters equal one centimeter; one centimeter equals 3/8 inch; one inch equals 2.5 centimeters.)

- **Size of the breast**—Some breasts may be too small in comparison to the size of the lump to give good cosmetic appearance when the lump is removed.

- **Location in the breast**—Tumors under the nipple sometimes may not give a suitable cosmetic look when the lump is removed.

- **Involvement of other structures**—The skin, muscle, chest wall, bone, or other organs.

- **General health**—Any treatment limitations due to her present health.

> *Anna had to decide what was the best surgical option for her. We discussed and researched the options at length, but she had to decide.*
>
> **—BRIAN CLUXTON**
> **SUPPORT PARTNER**

- **Appearance of mammogram**—To determine if the tumor is multicentric (lesions in more than one quadrant in the breast) or multifocal (two lesions in one quadrant of the breast). This is sometimes evidenced by microcalcifications (small calcium deposits) or mammographic abnormalities. The lesions may be too far apart, or require the removal of too much breast tissue, to give good cosmetic results with breast conservation.

- **Patient's desire for reconstruction**—The desired outcome for the reconstructive surgery (breast enlargement, reduction or to match the present breast size).

- **Surgery** that offers the best chance for a cure.

- **Surgery** that gives the best functional results for her arm and shoulder.

- **Surgery** associated with the fewest short and long-term complications.

- **Patient's** priorities regarding the surgery.

Each tumor must be evaluated in terms of its unique and specific features, as well as what surgery will be best for the patient. Some types of breast cancer may require neoadjuvant chemotherapy—chemotherapy treatments before surgery. This type of chemotherapy may be given to shrink a tumor to allow breast conservation (lumpectomy) with good cosmetic results.

LYMPH NODES

During the discussion about breast cancer surgery and treatment, the physician will talk about lymph nodes. Lymph nodes are small pea-like structures located very near the breast, under the arm, and near the collarbone and breastbone. They act as filters for the cells' waste, which is picked up by the lymphatic vessels and filtered through these tiny nodes. Cancer that leaves the breast is often found growing in the lymph nodes nearest the first nodes draining the tumor site.

Surgeons may remove some of the nodes so that the pathologist (a physician who studies cells for disease) can evaluate the nodes to see if there is any cancer found. The number of lymph nodes removed and evaluated varies according to the type of surgery. There are three levels of axillary nodes under the arm that drain the majority of the lymphatic fluid from the breast. These are the nodes that are checked during surgery, unless a procedure called "sentinel lymph node mapping and surgery" is used to identify the node closest to the tumor.

SENTINEL LYMPH NODE MAPPING AND SURGERY

Sentinel lymph node mapping is a new procedure that identifies the first nodes (sentinel) that receive lymphatic fluid from a cancerous tumor, thus identifying the lymphatic drainage pattern. The sentinel nodes are like the gatekeepers to the rest of the lymph nodes. Lymphatic fluid contains white blood cells, proteins, and fats that pick up the cellular waste of tissues and then the fluid flows through the nodes, which act as filters. Because this fluid passes through these nodes, the lymphatic system is a major route by which cancer spreads or metastasizes. Cancer cells can reach the lymphatic system and filter through the nodes where they multiply. They may pass also through the lymphatic system into the bloodstream. (See lymph node illustration on page 46)

Tumors may drain to different node chains, according to the position of the tumor in the breast. The procedure identifies the lymphatic chain and the nodes most likely to indicate whether cancer has metastasized to the regional lymph node area. This identification gives the surgeon and pathologist a reliable guide for more accurate node evaluation without removing a large number of nodes.

The procedure begins with an injection of a radiographic substance before going to surgery. Before surgery begins, the surgeon may inject a blue dye around the tumor site or areola; it is carried by the lymph fluid to the closest node(s) (sentinel). During surgery, a hand-held gamma-detection probe first identifies where the radiographic material has concentrated, showing the area for the surgeon to make the incision. If used, the blue dye helps the surgeon visually identify the node (there may be one or several) for removal. After surgery, the pathologist examines these nodes for cancerous cells. (Some surgeons may only use the dye.)

Sentinel node mapping improves the accuracy of selecting nodes to be removed surgically for evaluation to check for the spread of the cancer. It may also prevent unnecessary removal of nodes not in the lymphatic drainage field of the tumor. Reducing the number of nodes removed can greatly decrease the potential for future lymphedema (a swelling from lymphatic fluid accumulation in the arm, which can cause discomfort and is a lifetime risk) and the likelihood of an infection in the arm if any type of injury should occur.

BREAST CONSERVING SURGERY (LUMPECTOMY)

When possible, physicians strive to offer surgery that preserves the body image. However, breast-conserving surgery (lumpectomy) may not be appropriate because of:

- Pregnancy (unless delivery is within six weeks of cancer surgery)
- More than one primary tumor in another quadrant of breast
- Mammogram revealing suspicious scattered microcalcifications (small calcium deposits seen on film) in another area of breast
- Size of tumor (large tumor or breast too small in relation to size of the tumor will give poor cosmetic results)
- Prior radiation therapy to the breast or chest area (example: chest radiation for Hodgkin's disease)
- Collagen vascular disease (lupus, scleroderma, etc.)
- Severe chronic lung disease (not a candidate for radiation)
- Very large, pendulous breast (radiation oncologist determines patient's eligibility for radiation therapy)
- Evidence of remaining cancer in ducts surrounding tumor after surgery (if surgeon is unable to obtain clear surgical margins, this creates a high risk for recurrence)
- Restrictions on travel or transportation to clinic for daily radiation for five to seven weeks

LUMPECTOMY PROCEDURES

Lumpectomy procedures differ in the amounts of tissue removed based on the size of the tumor. Lymph node removal during breast-conserving surgery also varies. Ask the surgeon which of the procedures and the extent of tissue and lymph node removal she will need to have. Listed are the three basic types of breast conserving (lumpectomy) surgeries.

1. Partial or Segmental Mastectomy

The tumor, overlying skin, and an area of tissue around the tumor are removed in this surgery. A portion of the lining of the chest muscle under the tumor and some of the skin may also be removed. Lymph nodes may or may not be removed from under the arm by a separate incision, which is approximately two inches in length.

2. Tylectomy

The tumor and a wide area of tissue around the tumor are removed during surgery. Lymph nodes may or may not be removed by a second incision under the arm.

3. Lumpectomy

Lumpectomy removes the tumor and a small wedge of surrounding tissue. Lymph nodes may or may not be removed by a separate incision under the arm.

Incisions for these three breast-conserving procedures are very similar. The cosmetic appearance of the breast after surgery differs only according to the amount of tissue removed.

LUMPECTOMY

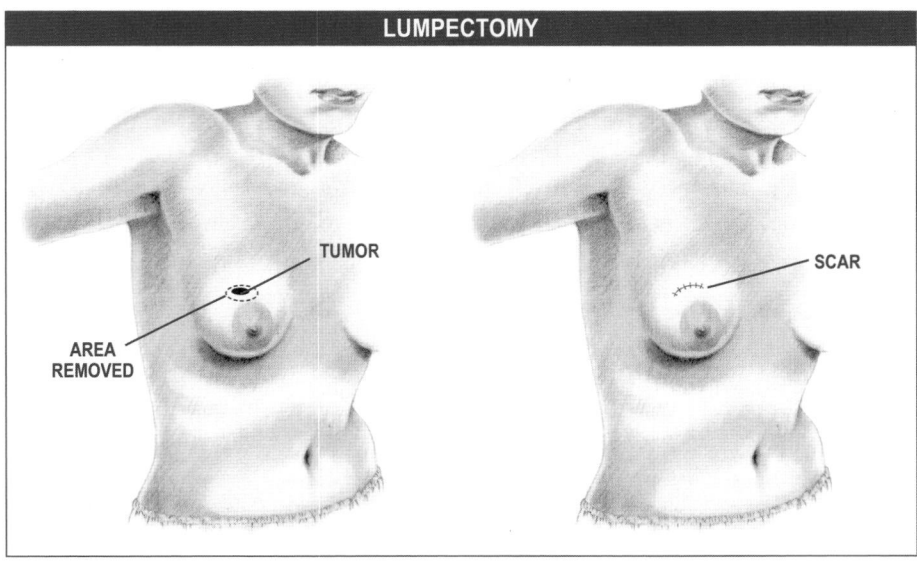

TUMOR

AREA REMOVED

SCAR

LUMPECTOMY AND AXILLARY NODE SCAR

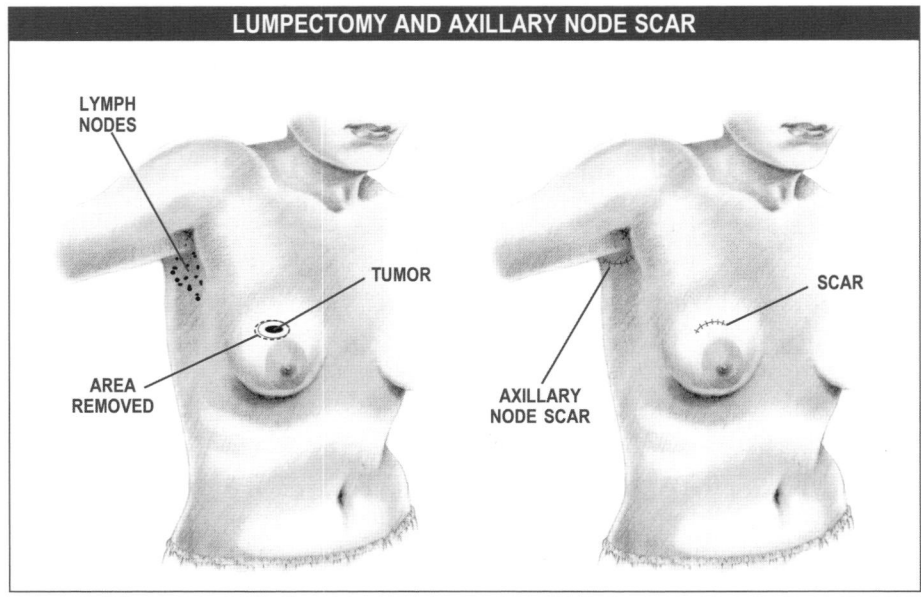

LYMPH NODES

TUMOR

AREA REMOVED

SCAR

AXILLARY NODE SCAR

MASTECTOMY

There are also several types of mastectomies. Your surgeon will tell your partner which procedures will be performed and how much tissue and lymph node removal is planned. The different mastectomies are defined below:

1. Modified Radical Mastectomy (Conservative or Limited)

A modified radical mastectomy removes the breast, nipple, areola, underarm lymph nodes, and the lining over the chest wall muscles.

You may hear the procedure referred to as a "total mastectomy with axillary dissection" which means that the entire breast and some or all of level one and two lymph nodes are removed. The chest muscles and pectoral nerves are not removed.

2. Full or Complete Modified Radical Mastectomy

A full modified radical mastectomy removes the breast, nipple, areola, all three levels of lymph nodes, small chest muscle (pectoralis minor), medial pectoral nerve, and the lining over the chest wall muscles.

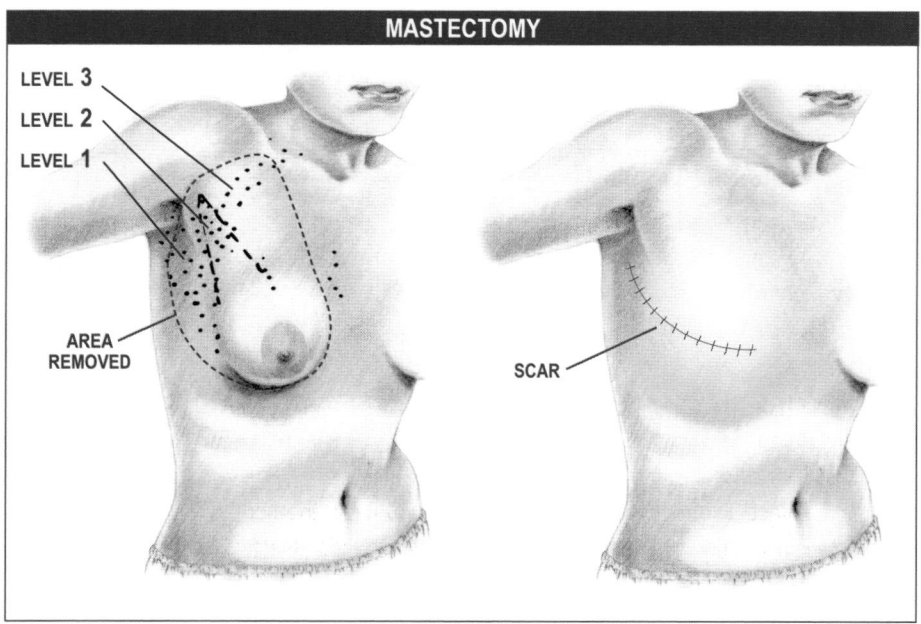

MASTECTOMY

LEVEL **3**
LEVEL **2**
LEVEL **1**

AREA REMOVED

SCAR

3. Total, Simple, or Prophylactic Mastectomy

This procedure removes the breast tissue, nipple, areola, and possibly some of the under-arm lymph nodes that are closest to the breast.

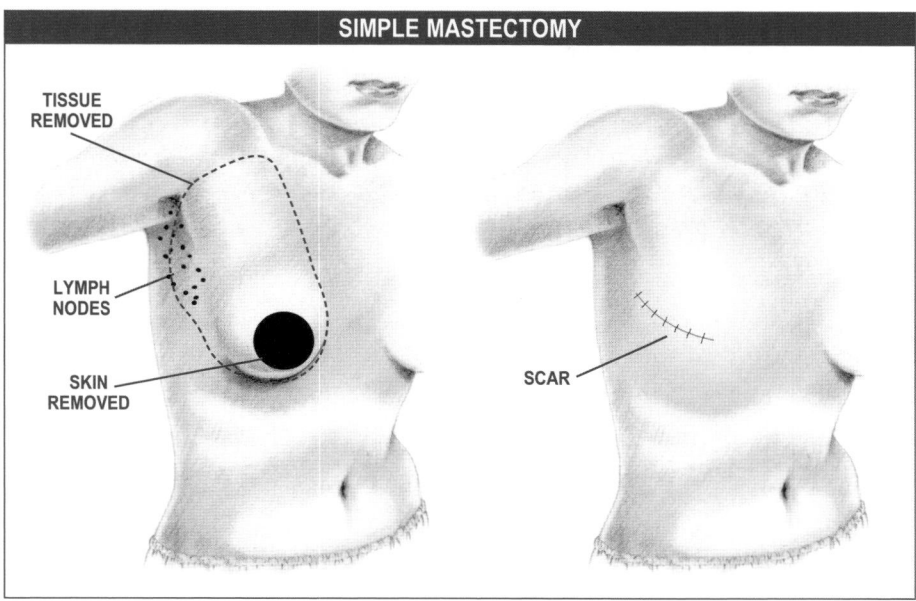

SIMPLE MASTECTOMY

TISSUE REMOVED

LYMPH NODES

SKIN REMOVED

SCAR

4. Skin-Sparing Simple Mastectomy

A skin-sparing simple mastectomy is a new procedure used when performing a simple or total mastectomy. The method removes the breast tissues from a circular incision around the areola (dark colored circle). The nipple, areola, breast tissues, nodes located near the breast tissues, and additional lymph nodes are removed according to the discretion of the surgeon. This procedure is often selected when reconstructive surgery is performed. The sparing of the skin allows reconstructive surgery to be performed with little need for a period of stretching of the skin. The sensitivity of the skin over the reconstructed breast remains intact. The reconstructive incision is made using the normal curve of the breast. This incision is not as visible because it is hidden under the fold of the breast and is concealed by the bra. The incision used to remove the breast is concealed by recon-struction of the nipple and areola.

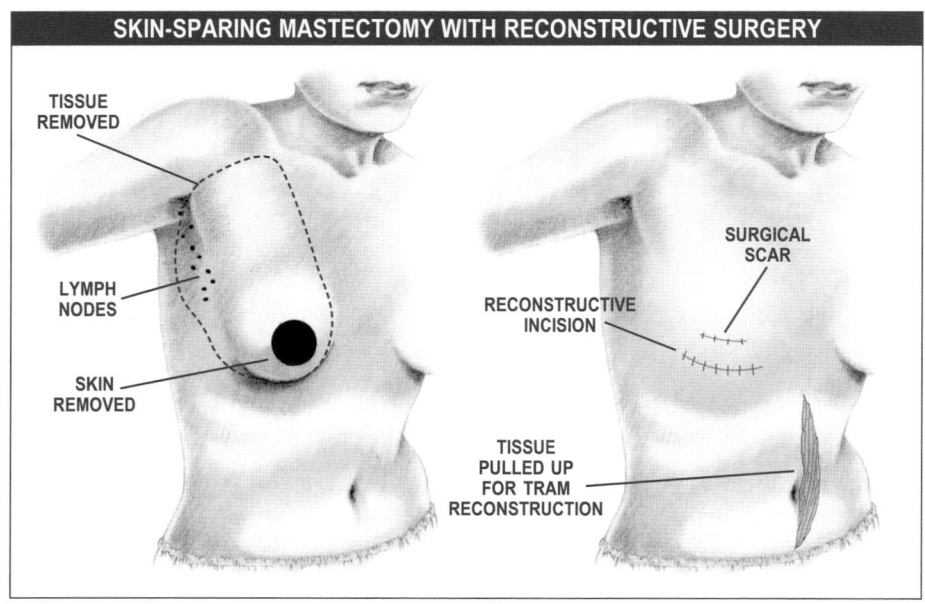

SKIN-SPARING MASTECTOMY WITH RECONSTRUCTIVE SURGERY

TISSUE REMOVED

LYMPH NODES

SKIN REMOVED

SURGICAL SCAR

RECONSTRUCTIVE INCISION

TISSUE PULLED UP FOR TRAM RECONSTRUCTION

LUMPECTOMY VERSUS MASTECTOMY

If the breast and tumor are within certain size limits, the surgeon may offer your partner the option of a lumpectomy (breast conservation) or a mastectomy. If she is given this option, the decision may be difficult for her. It needs to be a decision she makes in consultation with her physician, after careful review of the advantages and disadvantages of both procedures. (Remember, this option may not be available for some types of cancer.) It is imperative that she feels comfortable with the decision. Studies document that a lumpectomy, even if there is local recurrence, does not affect survival rate. However, the inconvenience may come from the necessity of having a second surgery. Note: The surgeon may wish to add additional variables to the following lists.

Lumpectomy Advantages

- Preserves body image by saving a large portion of the breast, usually the nipple and areola

- Patient is able to wear her own bras

- Slightly shorter hospitalization time, or surgery may be performed as an outpatient procedure; shorter recovery time

- May be psychologically easier to accept unless the fear of monitoring the remaining breast tissue (through breast self-exam, clinical exams, and mammography) is too frightening

Lumpectomy Disadvantages

- Risk of recurrence of cancer in remaining breast tissue

- Several weeks (usually five to seven) of radiation therapy to the remaining breast tissues

- Changes in texture, color (slight suntan)

- Sensation of feeling in the breast after radiation therapy may be slightly decreased

- Decrease in size of the remaining breast tissues after swelling decreases (following radiation treatments)

- Potential for chronic swelling or accumulation of fluid in the breast (breast lymphedema)

- Monthly breast self-exam becomes more difficult because of increased nodularity (lumpiness) from radiation therapy

- Possibility of future second lumpectomy or mastectomy if cancer recurs in the breast

Mastectomy Advantages

- Removes approximately 95 percent of all the breast gland; includes the nipple and areola, thus reducing local recurrence to the lowest degree

- Reconstruction of breast available using patient's own body tissue or synthetic implants

Mastectomy Disadvantages

- Body image changed because of the removal of the breast

- Need for prosthesis or reconstruction to restore body image

- Recovery time slightly longer than lumpectomy patients

If your partner is having problems deciding between a mastectomy and a lumpectomy, she may wish to speak with patients who have had the procedures. Your physician or your local American Cancer Society's Reach to Recovery program coordinator can provide her with the name of a volunteer who would be available to discuss her surgical procedure and decision-making experience. When considering a lumpectomy, a consultation with a radiation oncologist to discuss radiation treatments will provide additional insight to help your partner make an informed decision.

It is important to remember that a lumpectomy does not affect survival rate, even if there is a recurrence of the cancer. Each procedure offers an equal opportunity for survival. The inconvenience comes from the possibility of a second surgery if cancer recurs in the same breast.

RECONSTRUCTIVE SURGERY

Even though your partner may be losing a breast or a part of a breast through surgery, she has the option to have her body image restored through reconstructive surgery. Breast reconstruction has made a big difference, both physically and emotionally, for many women who have undergone breast cancer surgery. Some women choose to have reconstruction immediately following their initial breast surgery, while others wait until their treatments for breast cancer are completed. Some women choose to never have reconstruction, while others feel that reconstruction will help bring back their feminine silhouette, and allow them to avoid the necessity of wearing a prosthesis (breast form).

Some support partners are reluctant to discuss reconstructive surgery with their partners for fear of saying the wrong thing or having what they say misinterpreted. Clearly express to your partner that you accept her body image without reconstruction, but that you simply want her to explore any and all options that would be beneficial to her. In order for your partner to be able to maintain a sense of control over the cancer experience, she must be aware of all her options and able to choose those that meet her needs.

Many women have said that their partner's "I want you to do what you need to do" attitude granted them the freedom to discuss reconstruction without the pressure of feeling this procedure was necessary or important to their partner. If your partner expresses any desire to have her body image restored, she should discuss reconstruction with her surgeon prior to her breast surgery, thereby preserving all options for future reconstructive procedures. It is also advisable to consult with a reconstructive surgeon prior to surgery, even if she decides to have the procedure performed at a later date. Her surgeon or clinic can recommend reconstructive surgeons.

> *My wife was not given the choice of surgical options because of her tumor size. In some ways not having to make this decision was easier on us. However, the choice to have reconstructive surgery was not made easily. Helping my wife stand up for what she felt was best for her body took a lot of effort. I'm glad my wife sought my opinion, but the final decision had to be hers.*
>
> —AL BARRINEAU
> SUPPORT PARTNER

As with any optional surgical procedure, there are advantages and disadvantages to reconstructive surgery. The dilemma is in whether the advantages outweigh the disadvantages. Once a decision has been made to have reconstruction, the next step is for your partner to decide with her physician which type best suits her needs.

The breast may be reconstructed by placing an implant under the chest muscle. Implants may be composed of saline water, synthetic material, or a combination of both. Parts of a woman's own body tissue (autologous) may also be used. This tissue may be removed from her abdomen or back, or body fat from her buttocks may be used.

Insurance Coverage for Reconstruction

In 1998 a national bill, the Women's Health and Cancer Rights Act, was passed. It requires all health insurance providers who cover mastectomy procedures to also cover the cost of breast reconstruction and revision of the remaining breast if needed. This act covers:

- Reconstruction on the post-mastectomy breast (including immediate reconstruction)
- Procedure on the opposite breast to create symmetry between reconstructed breast and remaining breast (breast reduction, breast lift, etc)
- Breast prosthesis for women not choosing reconstruction (usually includes bras and replacement prosthesis; check with insurance providers on number of bras and frequency of replacement of prosthesis)
- Treatment of any complications caused by breast cancer surgery, including lymphedema (chronic swelling of surgical arm)

Reconstruction Type Criteria

- Physical makeup (size of breast, degree of sagging)
- Treatments given for cancer (Prior radiation therapy to the chest area may not allow some types of reconstruction)
- General health (example: smokers or diabetics may be poor candidates for some types of surgery)
- Desire to enlarge or reduce the other breast during surgery
- Personal goal and motivation for reconstruction

Age is not a factor for reconstruction. General health is, however, a primary factor. Health problems that may cause concern and limit surgical options are advanced diabetes mellitus, a recent heart attack or stroke, or a history of severe chronic lung disease. Smokers may also face limitations on the types of procedures available. However, only a physician can evaluate the health risks and determine if your partner is a candidate for reconstructive surgery. Some of the advantages and disadvantages of immediate and delayed reconstruction are listed below. Ask your reconstructive surgeon for additional observations.

Advantages of Reconstruction
- Retains her feminine body image
- Does not have to purchase or wear a prosthesis or special bras
- Can wear any clothing, including swimsuits and low-necked attire
- Can go braless
- Does not have the daily reminder of breast surgery by having to wear a prosthesis
- May adjust better psychologically to the disease

Disadvantages of Reconstruction
- Physical recovery from surgery will be longer if reconstruction is performed immediately or, if delayed, there is the need for additional surgery
- Increased potential for infection or surgical complications

IMMEDIATE VERSUS DELAYED RECONSTRUCTION

Advantages of Immediate Reconstruction
- One surgical experience, requiring only one anesthesia
- Lower cost than two separate surgeries
- Reduced recovery time because of only one surgical procedure
- Body image not as dramatic or unsettling as from a mastectomy alone without immediate reconstruction
- Psychologically, there may be some better adaptation

Disadvantages of Immediate Reconstruction
- More physical discomfort experienced and longer recovery time following surgery, when anxiety levels are at their highest (surgery time much longer if body tissues are used and only slightly longer if implants are used)
- Increased potential for infection or surgical complications, which could delay treatments

Advantages of Delayed Reconstruction
- Time to carefully study reconstruction methods and talk to patients who have experienced various procedures
- Time to carefully select a reconstructive surgeon and seek several consultations if needed
- Psychologically, less anxiety over cancer experience at time of reconstructive surgery
- No delay in treatments (chemotherapy or radiation) because of infection or surgical complications from surgery

Women with delayed reconstruction may be happier than women who have had immediate reconstruction because they lived with the change brought about by the mastectomy. (They have experienced the inconvenience of having to wear a prosthesis and the constant reminder of their disease; thus, their expectations were not as great as those who chose immediate reconstruction.)

Disadvantages of Delayed Reconstruction

- Need for a second major surgery

- Higher cost because of second major surgery (anesthesia, surgery room, etc.)

- Cost of purchasing a prosthesis and special bras

- Inconvenience of having to wear a prosthesis until surgery

- Unable to go braless or wear some low-cut clothing

- Sufficient time may have lapsed between surgeries requiring insurance deductibles to be met for a second time.

- Psychological distress from having to deal with an altered body image while waiting for reconstructive surgery

BREAST RECONSTRUCTION PROCEDURES

Tissue Expander Before Implant

This is the most common type of reconstructive surgery and provides good flexibility with breast size. The procedure may be done immediately, or later as outpatient or inpatient surgery. General anesthesia is usually used and the surgery takes approximately an hour to place the expander under the skin and pectoralis muscle. The expander is gradually filled with a saline (salt water) solution through a valve every few weeks for several months (3 – 6 months) to stretch the muscle and skin before the final implant placement. The skin and muscle are stretched slightly larger than the final implant. Additional surgery is required to remove the expander and position the permanent implant. Some women do not require the tissue expander before implant placement.

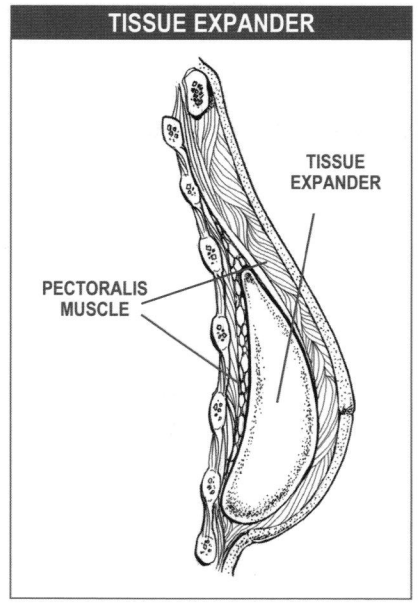

TISSUE EXPANDER

TISSUE EXPANDER

PECTORALIS MUSCLE

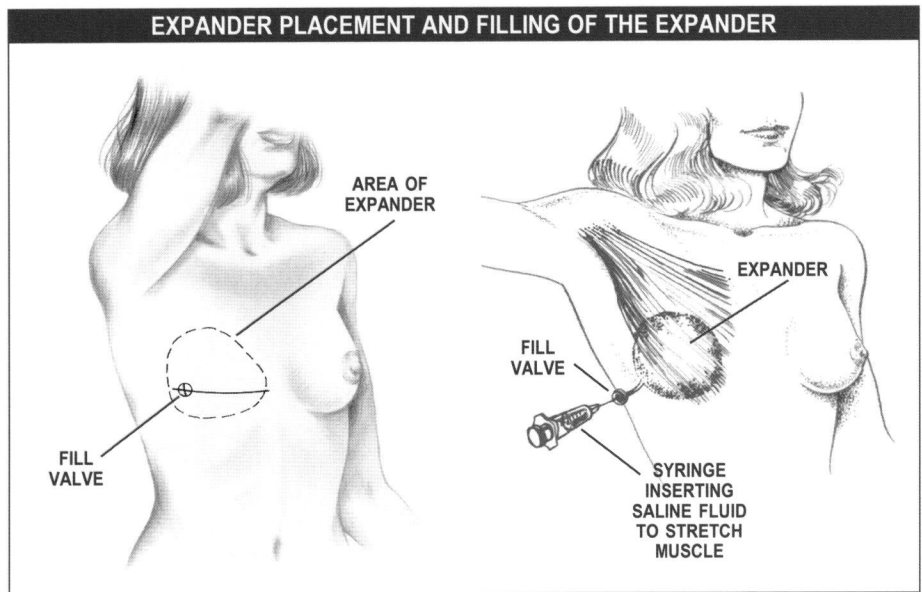

EXPANDER PLACEMENT AND FILLING OF THE EXPANDER

AREA OF EXPANDER

EXPANDER

FILL VALVE

FILL VALVE

SYRINGE INSERTING SALINE FLUID TO STRETCH MUSCLE

Implant (fixed volume implant)

A sack filled with silicone gel or saline fluid is implanted under the skin and chest muscle. Surgery is either outpatient or inpatient and lasts from one to two hours. Local or general anesthesia may be used. Silicone gel implants can be used only in clinical trials. Implants have very few surgical complications. The rates of such common surgical complications as seromas (collection of fluid under skin), hematomas (collection of blood under skin), and infection are relatively low.

Implant Disadvantages:

- Expander most often requires months to stretch out muscle and skin before body image is restored with implant placement
- Expander fill-valve may malfunction, requiring replacement
- Final implant may leak or rupture, requiring replacement
- Difficult to match a large remaining breast with implants
- Radiation therapy after implant placement increases risk of complications
- Capsular contracture risk (tissues around implant harden and distort its shape)
- Contracture may cause pain, as well visual change in shape
- Severe contracture may require removal of implant and placement of new implant

- Difficult to get reconstructed breast with implant to hang symmetrically on chest wall with opposite breast (implants cannot match natural droop of other breast)
- Implants will stay same size with weight gain or weight loss, unlike natural breasts
- Implants have a limited lifespan; they deteriorate and need replacement (potentially requiring more future surgical procedures)

Indications for Implants:
- Small to medium sized, with no drooping (ptosis)
- No previous radiation therapy to breast area
- Women not wanting additional scars
- Women who do not want longer, more complicated surgery
- Women in poorer general health or advanced age

AUTOLOGOUS TISSUE RECONSTRUCTIONS

Breast reconstruction using a woman's own body tissues (autologous) has many advantages, even with increased surgical complexity. A pedicle flap is a procedure that moves the tissues along with their own blood supply to the area. A free flap procedure cuts the tissues of the selected area from their blood supply and reattaches them through microsurgery to blood vessels in the breast area. Free flaps are the most complex of all reconstructive procedures, requiring a surgeon with expertise in microsurgery.

Autologous (Body Tissues) Reconstruction Advantages:
- Avoids many implant-related complications relating to future surgical procedures for revision or replacement of implant
- Autologous tissue implants have ample amounts of soft, warm and pliable tissues, more like normal breast tissue, unless a woman is extremely thin.
- Normal ptosis (drooping of breast) can be better matched.
- Normal inframammary crease (where the wire in an under-wire bra would be positioned) can be better matched to other breast
- Can add additional skin flaps to avoid having to stretch skin if mastectomy scar is tight
- Skin-sparing mastectomy procedure allows immediate reconstruction of the areola, avoiding a later surgical procedure.
- Post-surgical deformities or irregularities can be corrected with additional autologous tissues or an autologous flap.
- Donor sites (abdomen or hips) can have improvement in contour with reduction of body fat
- Lower cost over time because of fewer future complications and surgical revisions

- Volume and shape of autologous implants follow body weight changes
- Return of sensation is possible
- Breast feels warm when touched
- Provides solution for partial mastectomies or wide lumpectomies because of flexibility of tissues
- Preferred reconstruction if radiation therapy is to be part of cancer treatment

The most common sites of autologous tissue retrieval for reconstructions are:

1. **Abdomen:**
   TRAM (transverse rectus abdominis myocutaneous muscle)
   DIEP (deep inferior epigastric perforator)*

2. **Back:**
   LD (latissimus dorsi)
   TAP (thoracodorsal artery perforator)*

3. **Buttock:**
   Free superior or inferior gluteus
   S-GAP (free-superior gluteal artery perforator)*

*PERFORATOR FLAPS

Perforator flaps are recent refinements of conventional flaps where ***none*** of the underlying muscle is sacrificed. These procedures are relatively new. Ask your healthcare team if your reconstructive surgeons are skilled in these newer techniques.

Advantages of perforator flaps

- Preserving muscle decreases potential for future problems in donor site (weakness or restriction on activities)
- Preserving underlying muscle allows usual activities of daily living (sports, activities) as before surgery

Disadvantages of perforator flaps (DIEP, TAP, S-GAP):

- Reconstructive surgeon experienced in new procedure is needed
- Prolonged operating time because of complexity of procedure

ABDOMINAL TISSUES RECONSTRUCTION PROCEDURES

TRAM Flap (transverse rectus abdominis myocutaneous muscle)

The transverse rectus abdominis myocutaneous muscle (major stomach muscle) is moved to the breast area with fat and skin and is attached to form a breast. This procedure is most commonly called a tummy tuck. This is the most common type of autologous flap used at present and is excellent for women with additional abdominal fat. The transplanted tissue usually remains connected to its blood supply (called pedicle flap), but occasionally tissues and muscle will be cut loose (free flap) and reconnected by microsurgery. Inpatient surgery is required with general anesthesia, lasting three to five hours and requiring several days of hospitalization. The procedure is moderately painful, causing difficulty in standing up straight for several days or weeks because of the cut muscle. Drains may be left in place for several weeks. A scar is left on the abdomen where the flap is removed. Disadvantages are an increased weakness of the abdominal muscle and wall, limiting strength and making some activities difficult, along with an increased potential for hernia.

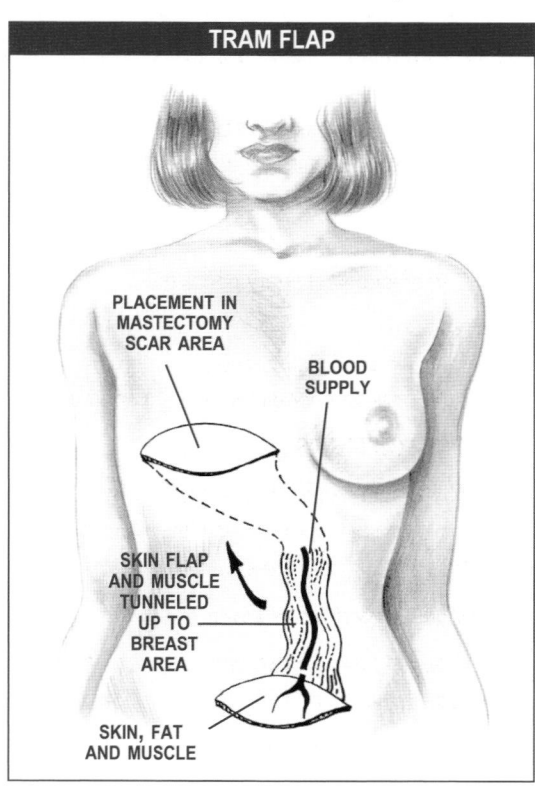

TRAM FLAP

PLACEMENT IN MASTECTOMY SCAR AREA

BLOOD SUPPLY

SKIN FLAP AND MUSCLE TUNNELED UP TO BREAST AREA

SKIN, FAT AND MUSCLE

DIEP (deep inferior epigastric perforator)

This procedure uses abdominal tissues without the abdominal muscle (rectus abdominis). The fat is harvested with local blood vessels (free flap, cut loose from local blood supply). Nerves can also be harvested along with the flap and used to restore sensation to the tissues when reattached in the breast area. Recovery time is reduced in this procedure compared to the TRAM flap because the muscle is not being moved, allowing earlier mobilization and return to normal activities.

BACK RECONSTRUCTION TISSUE PROCEDURES

Latissimus dorsi (back flap)

The back muscle, the latissimus dorsi, along with an eye-shaped wedge of skin are moved from the back and sewn in place on the breast area. The transplanted tissues are left attached to their original blood supply (pedicle flap). This is an inpatient procedure with general anesthesia lasting two to four hours and requires several days of hospitalization. The procedure is moderately painful, and a scar is left on the back. Drains may be left in place for several weeks. An implant, in addition to her own tissue, may be required to match the opposite breast because of the size of the latissimus muscle moved. Some procedures can be performed endoscopically (using special instruments under the skin) without leaving a scar on the back. This procedure is excellent for small, non-drooping breasts or for partial outer quadrant reconstruction.

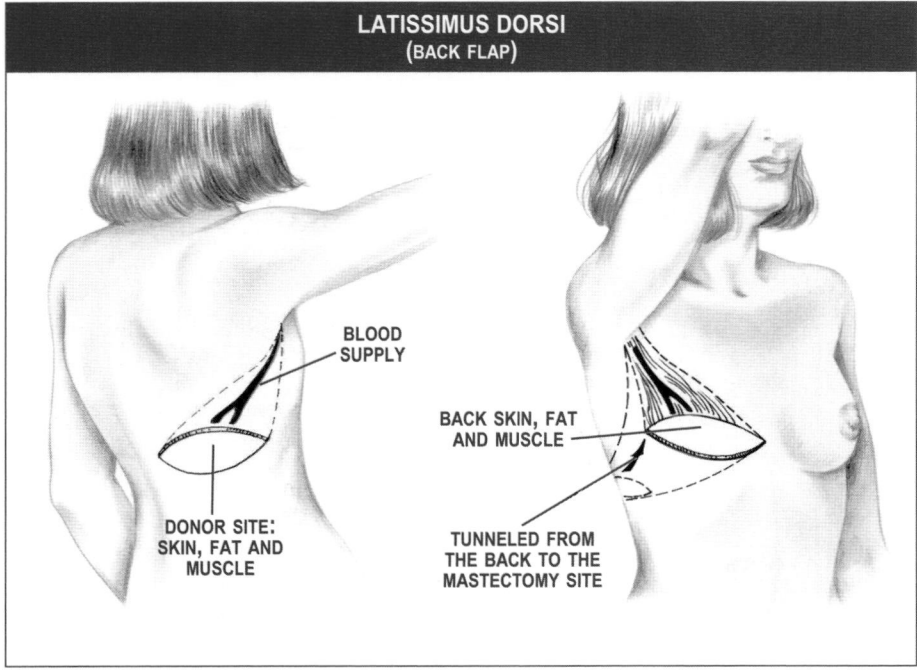

LATISSIMUS DORSI
(BACK FLAP)

BLOOD SUPPLY

BACK SKIN, FAT AND MUSCLE

DONOR SITE: SKIN, FAT AND MUSCLE

TUNNELED FROM THE BACK TO THE MASTECTOMY SITE

TAP (thoracodorsal artery perforator)

This procedure is an alternative to the latissimus dorsi flap; it does not move the muscle, but uses the fat of the upper and lower areas around the muscle. Because some women do not have a lot of additional fat in this area, it may not be the preferred procedure.

BUTTOCK TISSUES RECONSTRUCTION PROCEDURES

Inferior (lower) Gluteus (Buttock) Flap

This procedure uses a patient's own tissue from fat and muscle in the buttocks. The tissue is detached (cut free) from its blood supply and reattached to the breast area blood supply using microsurgery. This is an inpatient procedure that includes general anesthesia. Surgery can range from three to eight hours according to the degree of microscopic reattachment necessary. The scars on the buttocks are easily covered with underwear. Most women, except extremely thin ones, have tissue to spare.

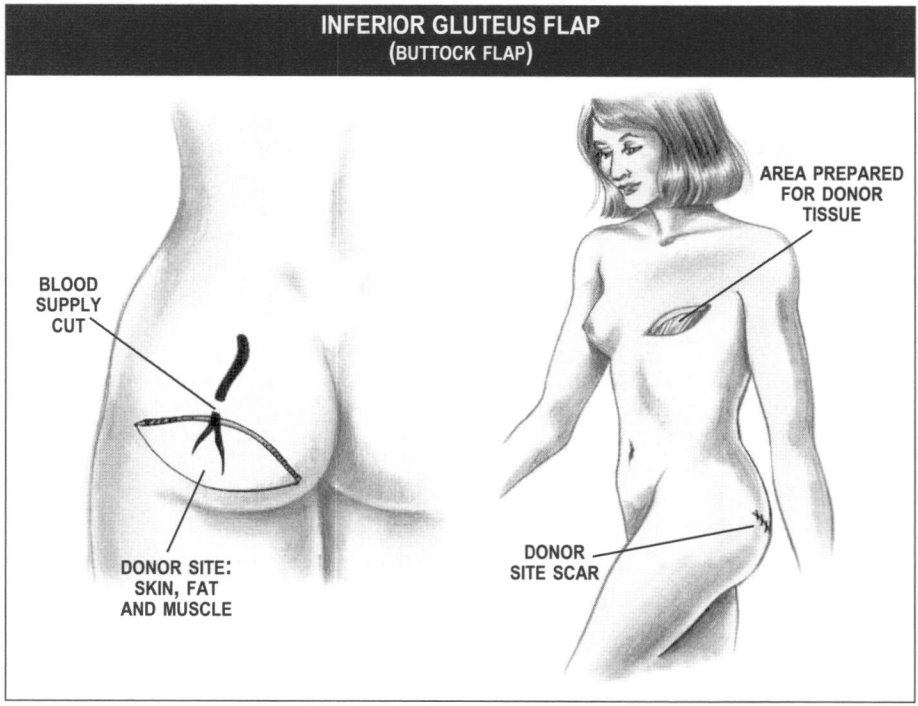

INFERIOR GLUTEUS FLAP
(BUTTOCK FLAP)

AREA PREPARED FOR DONOR TISSUE

BLOOD SUPPLY CUT

DONOR SITE: SKIN, FAT AND MUSCLE

DONOR SITE SCAR

FREE FLAP REATTACHMENT
(MICROSCOPIC PROCEDURE)

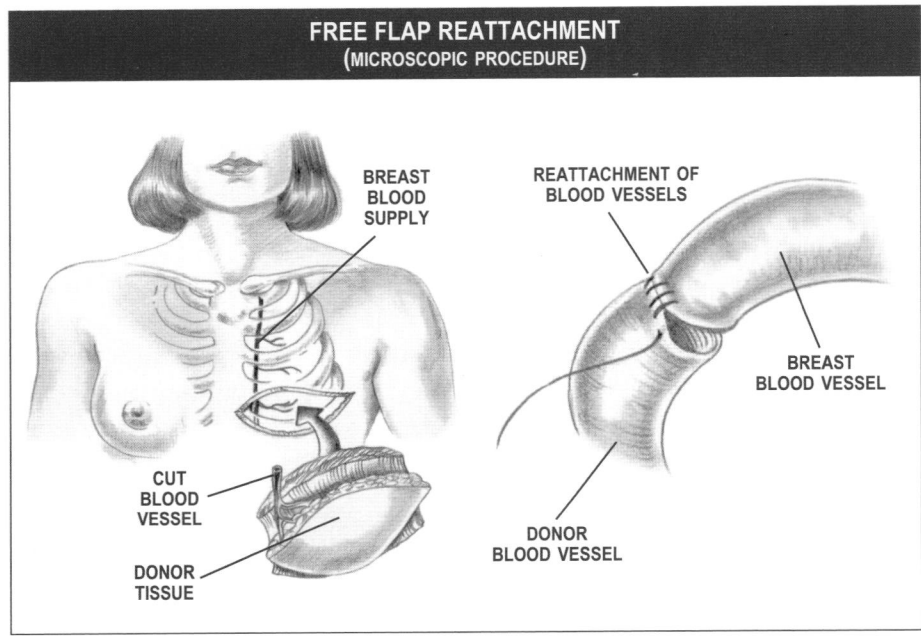

BREAST BLOOD SUPPLY

REATTACHMENT OF BLOOD VESSELS

BREAST BLOOD VESSEL

CUT BLOOD VESSEL

DONOR BLOOD VESSEL

DONOR TISSUE

FREE FLAP REATTACHMENT
(MICROSCOPIC PROCEDURE)

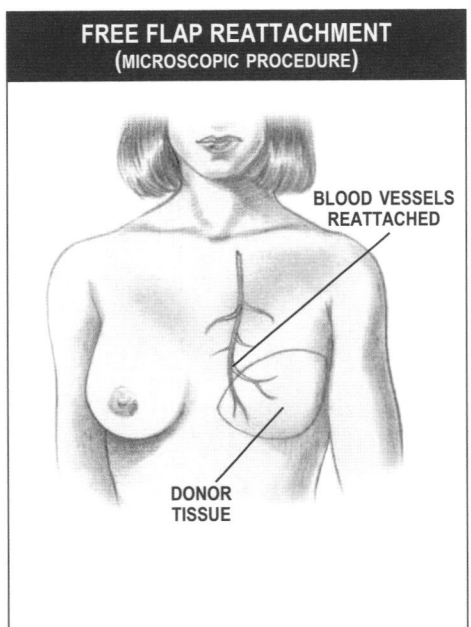

BLOOD VESSELS REATTACHED

DONOR TISSUE

S-GAP
(free-superior gluteal artery perforator)

This is an upgrade of the gluteus flap; it requires no muscle to be harvested and only the fatty tissue along with an artery for blood supply are moved to the breast and reattached using microsurgery. The tissue is removed from the upper portion of the buttocks (superior). This area has the potential to remove and transfer nerves to restore sensation to the new breast.

NIPPLE AND AREOLA RECONSTRUCTION

The nipple and areola are usually reconstructed from existing skin and fat on the breast itself, or occasionally from tissues removed from other areas of the body such as the groin. The skin is molded to form the shape of the nipple and attached to the breast mound. Areola reconstruction may be done by tattooing a dark pigmented color to match the other areola. Surgery is outpatient and pain is minimal. The procedure is usually performed about six months after reconstruction when breast symmetry is satisfactory. Some women choose not to have nipple and areola after breast reconstructive surgery.

RECONSTRUCTION AND BREAST CANCER DETECTION

Reconstruction does not alter the biology of breast cancer. It cannot cause an increase in local recurrence and does not compromise the ability to have adequate breast cancer treatment. Women often fear that reconstruction may hide or prevent the detection of cancer recurrence in the breast area in the future. Physicians report, however, that there is little difficulty in detecting early local recurrence because the breast implant is usually placed under the skin and beneath the chest wall muscles. Furthermore, there is no evidence of any kind that breast reconstruction causes cancer to grow or makes it recur. If a woman desires immediate reconstruction, it will not alter her disease-free interval or survival. These fears should not be of any concern in making a decision.

REMEMBER

SURGICAL AND RECONSTRUCTIVE DECISIONS NEED TO BE MADE BY ONLY YOUR PARTNER, AFTER SHE UNDERSTANDS THE ADVANTAGES AND DISADVANTAGES OF EACH PROCEDURE.

Complication Risks	Muscle Sparing (free-TRAM or DIEP)	Non-Muscle Sparing	Implants
Abdominal bulge or hernia	2 - 4%	5 - 10%	
Abdominal weakness	Virtually eliminated	30 - 60%	
Delayed healing	Less than 5% *	Less than 5% *	Less than 5% *
Premature removal related to rupture or capsular contracture or patient dissatisfaction			40% by 5 years
Free flap failure	3%		

*most common with previous radiation or smokers

COMPARISON OF BREAST RECONSTRUCTION PROCEDURES

Type	Advantages	Disadvantages	Indications	Contraindications
Tissue Expander and Implant	- Short surgical time - Low cost	- Multiple fillings of expander with saline - 2nd surgery for implant - Capsular contracture - Leakage or rupture	- Medium size breast (400 - 800 cc) - Lumpectomy defect - Tight skin from radiation therapy	- None - Previous radiation therapy may limit size
Implant: Saline or Silicone	- Short surgical time - One-step procedure - Lower cost	- Capsular contracture - Leakage or rupture - Autoimmune disease (>.5%)	- Small breast (400 - 600 cc)	- Thin skin flaps - Radiation therapy
Latissimus Dorsi Flap (Pedicle Flap) Muscle and Tissue	- Autologous tissue and muscle remain attached to blood supply - Small donor scar	- Minor muscle weakness - Potential seroma - Flap necrosis	- Small to medium size breast (400 - 800 cc) - Lumpectomy defect - Tight skin from radiation therapy	- None
TAP Thoracodorsal Artery Perforator (Free Flap) Tissues Only	- Autologous tissue with blood vessels - No muscle removed - Small donor scar	- Potential seroma - Flap necrosis	- Small to medium sized breast (400 - 800 cc) - Lumpectomy defect - Tight skin from radiation therapy	- Extremely thin women
TRAM Flap Transverse Rectus Abdominis Myocutaneous (Pedicle)	- Autologous muscle with tissues attached to local blood supply - Tummy tuck	- Scar on abdomen - Minor muscle weakness - Extended operative time - 6 - 12 wks. recovery - Abdominal wall hernia - Flap necrosis	- Mastectomy	- Previous abdominal surgery - Physical condition - Cigarette smokers (some physicians)
DIEP Deep Interior Epigastric Perforator (Free Flap)	- Abdominal tissues with blood vessels and nerves - Potential return of nerve sensations in area	- Additional scar on abdomen - Extended operative time from microscopic reattachment - Flap necrosis	- Mastectomy	- Previous abdominal surgery - Physical condition - Cigarette smokers (some physicians) - Extremely thin women
Inferior Gluteus Flap (Free Flap)	- Autologous tissues, muscle and blood vessels cut from lower buttocks	- Scar at donor site - 6 - 12 weeks recovery - Extended surgical reattachment time - Flap necrosis	- Mastectomy	- Cigarette smokers (some physicians) - Extremely thin women
S-GAP Superior Gluteal Artery Perforator (Free Flap)	- Autologous tissues, blood vessels, and nerves cut from upper buttocks - Potential return of nerve sensation	- Scar at donor site - Shorter recovery - Extended surgical reattachment time - Flap necrosis	- Mastectomy	- Cigarette smokers (some physicians) - Extremely thin women

FACING SURGERY TOGETHER

The period between diagnosis and surgery is an anxious and exhausting time for a woman and her support partner. Before her surgery, the patient will be required to have a pre-admission assessment at the hospital or clinic. The physical assessment, which usually takes one to two hours, may include a chest x-ray, blood work, electrocardiogram (EKG) and instructions for surgery. Though not physically imposing, it is often emotionally distressing, and a time most women find a supporting partner a great comfort. You and your partner should have the following questions answered during this assessment:

- What is the last time she can eat or drink before surgery?
- What regular medications should she take the day of surgery?
- What time do we need to arrive?
- Where do we park the car the day of surgery?
- To what area does the patient report?
- Will her surgery require an overnight stay?
- Should we bring in personal items or wait and take them to the room if admitted overnight?
- Where will I wait during surgery?
- How many people are allowed to wait in this area?
- Can I use my cell phone in the waiting area?
- What is the telephone number of the waiting room?

> *The hours in surgery were definitely the hardest time of the entire treatment period for me. I ended up walking around and around the hospital with my dad and my cell phone. I couldn't sit still, and it was good to have someone share my pain during this time.*
>
> **—BRIAN CLUXTON**
> **SUPPORT PARTNER**

- How long is a patient usually in surgery?
- How long is a patient usually in recovery?
- Who will be relaying information to me concerning her condition?
- Will I be able to speak with the surgeon after surgery?
- What are the visiting hours in the hospital, if admitted overnight?
- Am I allowed to stay in the room overnight if we so choose?

THE NIGHT BEFORE SURGERY

The night before surgery can be a very sad and stressful event for a woman. This is the last night with her body image intact. Some have to emotionally say goodbye to their breast as if it were an old friend. To ease her distress, plan to make this a special evening for both of you—a quiet early dinner at her favorite restaurant, or her favorite food at home. More important, however, is letting her know how important she is to you and that you are committed to be with her "no matter what comes." Give her space to work through this time in her own way with your silent support. While women will behave differently immediately prior to surgery, all appreciate a supportive, understanding partner committed to them.

THE DAY OF SURGERY

You have cried, fought the fears, looked for answers, and confronted difficult decisions. On the day of surgery, both of you will probably be drained emotionally and physically. However, surgery often brings a sense of relief to the patient, through knowing that the enemy has been removed and that she may now go forward.

Allow enough time to arrive at the hospital without rushing. This is undoubtedly an emotional time for both patients and their partners. Most women have a few tears left and are quietly withdrawn and visibly nervous about the surgery. Remember, what most women need is the presence of a support partner. There are no magical words or phrases to erase their fears, but your support will be what makes a difference.

> " *The early morning drive to the hospital was gloomy because of the cold and rain. We were both unusually quiet; each of us was locked in our own thoughts. This was the day we had dreaded, but now that it was here, we were ready to get it behind us. Just as we reached the hospital, the rain stopped and the skies cleared for a short time . . . assurance the sun would shine again for us.* "
>
> —AL BARRINEAU
> SUPPORT PARTNER

Many women have surgery as an outpatient and return home after a stay in a recovery unit. There they are monitored until all of their vital signs (blood pressure, respirations, heart beats per minute, etc.) are in normal range, they are not vomiting, and pain is controlled. After this they are released to go home. Be sure you understand all discharge instructions before she leaves the hospital or clinic. Read the instructions given to you by her nurse. Ask for clarification if needed. The patient may be awake and listening, but may not remember what is said because of the effects of the anesthesia. Ask for a name and telephone number that you may call if you have additional questions after you arrive home.

If admitted to the hospital, the patient will be drowsy from anesthesia when she arrives in her room. Many women confess that they were not emotionally up to having many visitors the first day. If your partner feels this way, ask the nurse to place a "no visitors" sign on the door so that she can rest, and either remove the telephone from the hook or answer the phone for her. Some women feel that this is a very personal time and would rather not have guests until they are feeling more in control of their emotions. Ask her what she would like for you to do to ensure she has adequate rest.

SAME-DAY DISCHARGE

You and your partner should have the following questions answered prior to discharge:

- How should pain be managed?
- What do we do if there is any nausea or vomiting?
- When and what can the patient eat?
- What regular medications can be resumed and when?
- If she has bulb drain(s) inserted during surgery to remove fluid accumulation at the surgical site, when and how should they be emptied? (Ask for a demonstration, if not previously given.)
- Should the amount of drainage be recorded? (Be sure you understand how to measure and record the amount.)
- To what extent can the surgical arm be used?
- Does the surgical arm need to be propped up on a pillow while she is lying down?
- Should the surgical dressing be changed before we return to the physician? (If yes, ask for detailed instructions and for supplies to take home.)
- What normal sensations should be expected to occur in the surgical area and arm?
- When can a bath be taken? What type of bath?
- When can her hair be shampooed?

- What symptoms need a physician's immediate attention? (Bleeding, increased pain, clogged drains, fever, etc.)
- When does an appointment need to be scheduled with the physician? (Do you call for an appointment or has one already been made?)

THE HOSPITALIZED PATIENT

While the time spent in the hospital following surgery is usually very short, most women have said they appreciate their partner's close presence. "I didn't want him to leave me. . . . Something inside of me wanted to say, 'Hold me and make it all right,'" admitted one patient. Spend as much time as possible with her. She may want you to spend the night with her. While this is not medically necessary, it may be psychologically comforting. Many women need extra closeness. This is the critical time when she needs to know that the change in her body image has not changed your love. Experience reveals that couples who are able to talk openly and assure each other of their committed love will emerge from the breast cancer experience with a stronger relationship.

GETTING THE FACTS

Following surgery, a new set of questions will surface. The best source for answers is your partner's physician and staff. Most physicians make their daily rounds to patients' rooms very early in the morning, before their office appointments begin. If possible, arrange to be in your partner's room at this time to ask the physician your questions. Make a list (sample above) so you do not forget what you need to ask. If your list of questions will require an extended amount of time to be adequately answered, schedule an appointment with the physician at the office. The nursing staff is also available to answer many of your questions. Physicians often have a nurse who is trained to provide information for the patient and her family.

PREPARATION FOR VIEWING THE SCAR

For patients staying overnight in the hospital, physicians often remove the surgical dressing and look at the incision the morning before the patient leaves the hospital. Ask if this is the policy of your physician. Others who have outpatient surgery will have their first dressing change the day of their first return visit to the physician.

I can tell you from experience, viewing the surgical scar is often one of the most difficult tasks for some women or their partners. Nudity after breast surgery is a difficult issue for many women. This event may threaten an intimate relationship more than any other aspect of the breast cancer experience. In fact, there are some women who have never allowed their partner to see them nude after surgery. Twenty years after surgery, some women are still dressing and undressing in the dark or behind closed doors. It never became emotionally easier to share their new body image with their partner.

Because viewing the surgical scar can be a roadblock to restoring an intimate physical relationship, planning before surgery to view the scar together as early as possible removes this potential barrier. For some, it will never be easy. Talking about it before surgery and planning together helps start the recovery process.

Deciding in advance to view the incision when the physician changes the dressing works well for many couples. The physician is there to answer any questions and explain how the scar will change as it heals. As a support partner, it is also helpful to watch as a nurse applies a new dressing, in case a dressing would need to be changed at home. It is very difficult to change a dressing on your own chest. This is a task that a support partner can perform that will be helpful. It also serves to promote the growth of acceptance and emotional bonding as a couple.

If your partner is having difficulty, don't force the issue of when, but encourage her to allow you to share this as soon as she feels she can.

> *I was so grateful a surgical procedure could be performed to rid her body of the cancer. However, my mate had to make peace with her scar before she allowed me to see it. This took several days. We had been able to communicate about it from the beginning and that helped us both. I was prepared for the scar and new body shape to be much worse than it was. I really didn't mind the way she looked. Her breast did not make her the person I loved, and the loss of her breast would not stop my loving her. The scar seemed easier for me to accept than for her—but then, it was her body that was involved and not mine. She needed my assurance that this would not change our relationship.*
>
> **—AL BARRINEAU**
> **SUPPORT PARTNER**

FIRST SCAR VIEWING

Your partner will be looking closely at your eyes to see your response at the first viewing of her new body image. To prepare for the viewing, ask your physician or nurse to show you pictures of what the incision will look like. They will share pictures and drawings with you that will help you know what the area will look like. This allows preparation on your part to reduce the potential for looking surprised or frightened when you see her surgical scar the first time. Your first response is very important and will always be remembered. Your response can serve as a foundation for her own personal acceptance by her new body image.

REMEMBER

ACCOMPANYING YOUR
PARTNER TO HER
PRE-ADMISSION WORKUP IS
PSYCHOLOGICALLY COMFORTING.

THE NIGHT BEFORE SURGERY IS A
HIGHLY EMOTIONAL TIME
FOR MOST WOMEN.
CAREFUL, SENSITIVE
PLANNING CAN MAKE IT
EASIER FOR BOTH OF YOU.

MOST WOMEN NEED EXTRA
PHYSICAL CLOSENESS PRIOR TO
AND IMMEDIATELY
FOLLOWING SURGERY.

ASK FOR CLEAR
DISCHARGE INSTRUCTIONS.

DISCUSS WITH YOUR
PARTNER WHEN TO VIEW THE
SURGICAL AREA AND DO NOT
ALLOW IT TO BLOCK AN
INTIMATE RELATIONSHIP.

PREPARE FOR THE VIEWING BY
LOOKING AT SURGICAL DRAWINGS
OR PICTURES OF WHAT THE SCAR
MAY LOOK LIKE.

COUPLES THAT MANAGE BEST WITH
THIS ISSUE PLAN TO GET THIS
POTENTIAL SEXUAL ROADBLOCK
BEHIND THEM AS EARLY AS
POSSIBLE.

Dr. Charles Carver, a professor of psychology at the University of Miami in Florida, conducted a study of 240 breast cancer surgical patients involved in long-term relationships and its impact on their relationships with their partners. Couples were followed for one year past surgery. Data from the study reported that, "How a husband reacts to his wife's breast cancer scars can have a big impact on her sense of femininity and the overall health of the couple's relationship. The less breast cancer patients felt their partners were bothered by their surgical scars, the more likely they were to report feeling feminine and attractive."

One woman fondly recalled, "He looked at my scar and said, 'This will always serve as our reminder of how lucky we were to be spared your life. . . . Your breast for your life. Thank God it was a breast, and I still have you. What a deal!' Later, as I looked at my scar, I remembered what he had said, and it was easier for me to accept." Giving special meaning to the new scar early helped this couple avoid a potential problem.

Dr. Carver concluded from the study, "Overall, the more the women saw their partners as affectionate and emotionally involved after the surgery, the more satisfied they were with the relationship."

RESUMING COMMUNICATIONS...
WHAT DO I SAY?

ome support partners find it painful to talk about the surgical experience. "Losing my breast was not nearly as hard as losing my mate emotionally . . . He wouldn't talk about it after surgery," lamented one patient. "He stayed away from home except when he was eating or sleeping . . . When I tried to talk about my cancer experience, he just looked at me and would not say anything."

Communicating after breast surgery can be difficult for both the patient and the partner. Many find it hard to express their thoughts, fearful that they may hurt the other's feelings or "lose it emotionally." Barriers are often erected to prevent communication from occurring. The most common barrier is emotional withdrawal—silence.

Emotional seclusion becomes a safe retreat. The workplace or hobby often becomes a safe place to hide. Being absorbed in work often becomes the antidote for emotional pain. However, this withdrawal or silence may be perceived as rejection or withdrawal of your love. This may lead to anger from your mate—expressed or internalized—and can eventually lead to depression. This emotional trauma can usually be avoided through early, honest communication. You must talk! You must listen! While painful at first, it is necessary for an emotional recovery from breast cancer. Communicate your feelings to each other—anger, fear, and sorrow–whatever they may be. Don't push or force the issue, but realize that not talking about cancer may be as dangerous to a relationship as cancer is to the physical body.

Understand that she needs to feel free to express her thoughts without judgement from you. Patients know there are no perfect answers; they just need to talk. Many times women need to say the same thing over and

> " I really had to work hard to listen and not try to 'fix it.' "
>
> —BRIAN CLUXTON
> SUPPORT PARTNER

over, so the best advice is just to listen. Do not be afraid of hearing about her fears and feelings, or seeing her tears. Remember, tears are a sign that she is in touch with reality and is successfully grieving her loss. Your tears are not a sign of weakness and will not weaken your relationship. One woman shared, "For the first time in my life, I saw the tears in his eyes as we talked about my surgery, and I knew without a doubt that he felt what I was feeling. Somehow from that point on I knew we were going to make it together." Tears have a language of their own and often say what we could never verbalize. They prove to the other that we are emotionally in touch with their pain and share their sorrow.

Communicating is difficult for some. They feel as if they don't know what to say. Spoken under stress, words often become even more powerful and may even be misinterpreted. For this reason, it is helpful to review some things that may prevent you from effectively communicating your love and concern for your partner.

Being stressed over the future is a normal part of a cancer diagnosis. Needing to share concerns and worries is a vital part of coming to terms with natural fears and helps her sort out options. Helping her feel comfortable talking with you requires that you listen attentively and know how to ask questions that give her permission to continue to share her real fears and feelings. Your goal is to solicit information from her.

You can do this by asking open-ended question such as: "Tell me how you feel about ____." "Share your thoughts about this decision with me." These open-ended questions allow the doors of communication to be opened. Some women need this verbal invitation to share their thoughts and feelings. They are not going to talk until given permission and they know that they have a safe place to share without someone being judgmental or critical of their innermost thoughts and fears.

> *After surgery she needed to talk and talk. I had never known her to talk so much. She drew comfort from my response, even when it was only a nod of agreement. Listening to her fears, her hopes, and sharing her tears was what she wanted most. At times, I didn't want to hear what she was saying. I wanted to hide in the newspaper or television, but I knew she needed me. I'm glad I took the time to listen.*
>
> —AL BARRINEAU
> SUPPORT PARTNER

Statements and open-ended questions that encourage and promote good communication are as follows:

- Tell me about what happened to you.
- Go on . . . tell me more.
- Give me an example of what you mean when you say . . .
- Describe that further for me.
- Describe how you felt when that happened.
- Please explain that to me, I want to better understand how you feel.
- Explain the details in the order that you remember them.
- Help me to understand what you mean when you say that.
- How important was that to you?
- What do you think the reason was for that to occur?
- What do you see as the problem?
- What do you mean when you say that?
- If I heard you correctly, you said (repeat statement).
- Let me restate what I heard you say.
- Is this what you were saying/feeling?
- What would you do if this situation occurs again?
- What would you want to happen if this situation occurs again?

Listed on the following pages are barriers to communication along with helpful and non-helpful responses. Read them carefully to see if there are any areas that may improve your communication skills with your partner.

THERAPEUTIC COMMUNICATION GUIDELINES

BARRIERS	NOT HELPFUL	HELPFUL
Giving Advice	Why don't you ___?	Have you considered ____ at this time?
	If I were you, I would ___.	What do you think would work best for you?
	You need to _____.	A good option to think about is _____.
		Some women find _____ helpful.
False Reassurance	Don't you worry!	What worries you most about this situation?
	Everyone feels like that.	Tell me what you are feeling.
	Things look worst before they get better.	This must be a very hard time for you. How are you handling this emotionally?
	This will be a piece of cake.	You seem to have all of the qualities it takes to do well during treatment.
Changing the Subject	Let's talk about that later.	That sounds important, tell me more.
Judgmental Attitude	You are wrong about that.	You understand this differently than I do. How do you see the situation?
	Don't think like that!	Tell me what you are thinking now.
	That's not a good decision when you have cancer.	I may not agree with your decision, but I understand where you may be coming from.
Direction Giving	This is the way you should do this.	Which of these ways do you think would work best for you?
	You need to / must follow the instructions.	Let's look at different options you have. How would you handle the situation?
Emotionally Charged Words	Your doctor/nurse/mother/child makes you very angry.	How do you feel about what he/she did?
	I'd tell them to mind their own business if they ask.	Do you mind people being inquisitive about your illness?
	Your doctors should not say that to you!	What do you think about what he/she said to you?

BARRIERS	NOT HELPFUL	HELPFUL
Challenging	You can't do that yet!	It sounds like you think you may be well enough to ____ now. Do you think that is wise?
Stereotyping Comments	You look chipper!	Gee, you're smiling a lot today, does that mean you're feeling better?
	Things always look better in the mornings.	How hard is it for you to keep going during chemotherapy?
	No pain, no gain!	Dealing with pain is tough, how are you handling all of this?
	Bald is beautiful you know!	Hair loss is the hardest side effect for many people during treatment, how are you feeling about it?
	It is better to lose a breast than to lose your life.	The loss of a breast must be very hard to deal with, how are you feeling about your surgery?
	Breasts aren't necessary for good sex.	Some women have trouble feeling sexy after breast surgery, how are you feeling?
Value Statements	You just need to have faith.	I know this is hard, this is testing my faith too.
	Relax, God is in control.	Sometimes its hard to feel God's presence.
	You just need to pray and let this fear go.	Can we pray about this together?

THE MAGICAL COMMUNICATION SKILL

There is a type of communication that works magic without words, and this is non-verbal body communication. You can convey much by the way you physically respond to her during this time. Instead of words, use your body language to speak. Hold her hand; make direct eye contact; place your hand on her shoulder; pat her back; sit or lie close to her; lean forward when she is speaking; wink at her when you catch her eye in public; seek out her presence in a crowd, to let her know you are aware of her. There are numerous other ways you can convey your love without saying a word. A large part of communication is body language. Your body language can be a very powerful source of comfort and communication during this time of stress. It can convey your love and concern when you can't find the right words.

REMEMBER

COMMUNICATION IS EVEN
MORE ESSENTIAL AFTER
BREAST CANCER.

WOMEN LISTEN INTENTLY
TO WHAT YOU SAY
(AND DON'T SAY)
AND OBSERVE YOUR
BODY LANGUAGE.
BE CAREFUL NOT TO SEND
MIXED MESSAGES.

LISTENING IS AN IMPORTANT
PART OF COMMUNICATION.
LET HER TALK.
TALKING CAN
BE THERAPEUTIC.

The other part of the magic is learning to read her body language. Carefully observe her body language for signs of personal need:

- Look at her eyes for signs of distress
- Frowns for signs of disapproval
- Squinting of eyes for a desire to better understand
- Tears for signs of feelings of loss, helplessness, or aloneness
- Questioning stares as a need for additional information
- Slumped posture as a sign of discouragement
- Closing of eyes as a sign of discouragement or emotional withdrawal
- Failure to make eye contact, as a sign of desire to avoid a person
- Repetitive movement of arms and legs, or tapping of fingers as a sign of high anxiety

When you observe her body language, you can then clarify her needs with statement such as, "I feel that you may be tired (upset or concerned or confused) about _____, is this an accurate observance?" Observing her body language and verbalizing these observations conveys absolute recognition of her needs and then allows her to verify or communicate previously unspoken concerns.

Effective communication and support from a partner is one of the best tools for recovery. In fact, women in our focus groups rated their need for support as high as their need for medical treatment during breast cancer. Direct, sensitive communication between partners in a caring non-judgmental manner enables a healthy acceptance and problem-solving approach, facilitating the emotional recovery from breast cancer.

During a crisis, communication skills become extremely important. Your mate faces a multitude of decisions, changes and losses at this time. She is forced into stressful situations. Your ability to allow her to express her feelings in an atmosphere of understanding rather than judgement can powerfully influence her ability to cope. Effective communication skills help avoid creating additional stress as well as resolving situations once they arise. Remember that communication is not just talking, but also the art of listening well.

When she talks:

- Look directly into her eyes.

- Turn off the television or put down the paper.

- Don't constantly look around to see what others are doing.

- When she has stated what she needed to say, clarify what she meant if you are uncertain.

- Ask opened ended questions to encourage her to tell you more.

- Respond with statements that reflect your respect for her opinions, fears or questions.

If something she says upsets you:

- Stop, take a deep breath.

- Think about "why" you are upset about what she said.

  - Do you feel compelled to stop her hurt and make everything all right?

  - Do you feel a need to "win" this point of difference?

  - Do you feel that you need to set her straight on the facts?

  - Do you feel that if she just did what you told her to do there would not be a problem?

  - Are you afraid to show any sign of weakness?

  - Do you feel you just don't want to hear all of this again?

- Determine why her words created stress in you and then carefully choose how you respond.

Remember that choosing to be an effective support partner is a choice that you make constantly. Often this requires new skills of communication. From her point of view, I would like to share with you the reading.

I NEED A HEART TO TALK TO

I need to talk.
And all I ask is that
you listen to me.

Somehow, when my heart
pours forth its thoughts,
fears and worries, they lose some of
their power over me.

When you stop me with
"you shouldn't feel that way" or
"don't say that" advice,
you push the power of their terror back
deep into my heart.

Where once again in the dark of night,
the power of their terror engulfs
my spirit with fear and confusion.

You say you want to help.
I just need a heart to listen to me
when I need to talk.

I don't need "head advice,"
I just need a heart to intimately
share the moment.

I need a heart that feels
for a few seconds, what I feel.

I need a heart that shares my
sorrows, with compassion.

I need a heart that recognizes
my fears as my own struggle
to face the unknown.

I need a heart of trust, so that when I
pull out the terror inside of me,
I feel that it will be allowed to
dissipate in the clean air
of another caring heart.

When all is said and done,
what I am asking for is your heart of
understanding when I talk.

I don't need any more "head advice."

Somehow, heart listening is a
more powerful medicine to my spirit.

— JUDY KNEECE

95

SILENT PRESENCE

SPEAKING TO THOSE WHO WERE
SERVING AS A SUPPORT
PARTNER TO SOMEONE WITH CAN-
CER, DR. SPIEGEL
PARAPHRASED THE OLD
ADMONITION,
"DON'T JUST STAND THERE,
DO SOMETHING," TO
"DON'T JUST DO SOMETHING,
STAND THERE,"
SIGNIFYING THAT SOMETIMES THE
GREATEST GIFT WE CAN GIVE IS
OUR SILENT PRESENCE. AT TIMES,
THERE ARE NO "GOOD" WORDS
THAT CAN BE SAID. THE PATIENT
JUST NEEDS US TO STAND ALONG
BESIDE THEM AND SILENTLY
SHARE THEIR SORROW.

— DR. DAVID SPIEGEL

UNDERSTANDING THE PATHOLOGY REPORT

Most treatment decisions will be based on information from the biopsy and surgical pathology reports, taking into consideration the patient's age, menopausal status, and general health. Pathology reports are often very technical, making them difficult for a layperson to understand. Yet, the pathology report contains most of the vital information on which treatment decisions are based. Years ago, pathology reports were kept secret from patients and their families. Today, many physicians feel it is helpful if patients and their families understand the diagnosis to the degree with which they feel comfortable. The pathology report may help a patient understand why a particular treatment protocol is needed and why it may be unlike someone else's. This is often accomplished through the physician's explanation of what the report reveals. Because this explanation may be hard to understand without a lay interpretation of the meaning of the terms used, the terms are included in this chapter.

You may find it helpful to familiarize yourself with the terms you may hear during discussions about treatment decisions. While it is not essential that you or your partner understand all of the following information, you may find it helpful as a future reference if needed. Some pathologists are happy to explain a report in detail.

> *Surgery produced a lot of stress and anxiety. Then came another stressor, the final pathology report. This was the report that contained the secrets of what was in her body and would direct her future treatment. Yet, it was very difficult for me as a layperson to understand. The answer was in having a doctor explain the report in terms we could understand. So, don't let it confuse you: ask a physician to explain it to you.*
>
> **—AL BARRINEAU**
> **SUPPORT PARTNER**

There will be two pathology reports. The first will be from the biopsy and the second from the surgery. Surgical decisions are based upon the preliminary biopsy report. Information from this report is combined with the final surgical pathology report to determine the stage of the cancer and the need for further treatments of chemotherapy, radiation therapy, or hormonal therapy.

HOW THE TUMOR IS ASSESSED

When the tumor is removed from the breast, it is sent to a pathology laboratory. There, a pathologist (a physician who specializes in diagnosing diseases from tissue samples), analyzes the biopsy sample and issues a pathology report to your physician. This report helps the physicians determine if additional treatment is needed. If treatment is needed, the pathology report is used by the oncologist (cancer specialist) to develop a treatment plan for the patient's cancer, based on the findings in the report. The report provides information on the following aspects of the tumor, which are explained later in more detail:

- type of breast cancer
- margins
- characteristics of the cancer
- tumor grade
- proliferation markers
- other diagnostic tests
- tumor size
- shape
- node status
- prognostic tests
- hormone receptor assay test results

COMMON TYPES OF BREAST CANCER

Infiltrating or invasive ductal ....(approximately 52%)

In situ ductal or intraductal ....(approximately 21%)

Invasive or infiltrating lobular ....(approximately 5%)

In situ or noninvasive lobular ....(approximately 2%)

Medullary ....(approximately 6%)

Mucinous or colloid ....(approximately 3%)

Paget's disease, intraductal or in situ ....(approximately 1%)

Paget's disease, invasive or infiltrating ....(approximately 1%)

Cancers occurring in 1 percent or fewer patients: Tubular, Papillary, Adenocystic, Inflammatory, Scirrhous, Apocrine, Squamous.

There are various other rare types of breast cancer as well as combinations of the above types.

TUMOR SIZE

Tumor size is the largest dimension of the tumor. Results are reported in centimeters (cm) or millimeters (mm).

10 mm equals 1 cm.

1 cm equals 3/8 inch.

1 inch equals 2.5 cm.

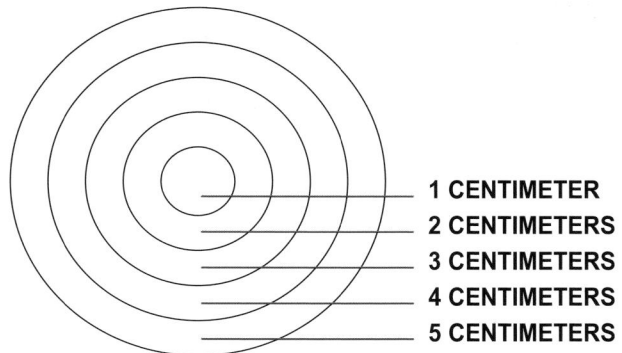

1 CENTIMETER
2 CENTIMETERS
3 CENTIMETERS
4 CENTIMETERS
5 CENTIMETERS

MARGINS

Margins describe the area surrounding the tumor, or if the entire tumor was removed, and tells how the margins relate to the tumor. If the tissue surrounding the tumor had no evidence of cancer cells, the terms used to describe the margins will be "clear," "clean" or "uninvolved." If cancer is found in the margins the descriptive terms may be "involved" or "residual cancer." If the pathologist is unable to make a definite statement, the term "indeterminate" may be used.

SHAPE OF TUMOR

The report may also describe the shape of the tumor as round or spherical (well-circumscribed) or of an irregular shape (stellate, poorly circumscribed). The more irregular the shape of a tumor, the higher the potential is for it to be aggressive or likely to spread.

CHARACTERISTICS OF CANCER

The cancer will either be in situ or invasive. (Refer to illustrations in Chapter 9)

In Situ Cancer—Normal ducts and lobules are lined with one or more layers of cells in an orderly pattern. Cancer is considered "in situ cancer" when it develops and grows but does not break through the wall where it began and remains in the duct or lobule.

Invasive (Infiltrating) Cancer—Cancers that have broken through the wall of the duct or lobule and have begun to grow into surrounding tissues in the breast are called invasive, or infiltrating.

NODE STATUS

If surgery included lymph node removal, the report will state how many nodes were removed, a description of the area from which the nodes came, and how many nodes tested positive with cancer cells.

GRADING OF TUMOR

The grading of cells involves a microscopic examination describing the degree of change from the original parent cell. This grading determines aggressiveness. Your pathology report may or may not report grades of differentiation. Tumors are classified as:

Grade 1: Well differentiated tumors—Less than 25 percent of the cells are abnormal. Approximately 75 percent or more of the cells are very similar in appearance to the parent cell (original cell) from which they evolved. They look similar, like sisters. Usually least aggressive.

> *In the beginning, I thought my wife would die. I thought breast cancer was a death sentence. When the physician explained the particulars of her pathology report, it gave us a renewed hope that our dreams for the future could still be realities. We were told the factors that were significant for her prognosis. Several things in the pathology report helped us know that her cancer was part of a large disease, but was also uniquely hers. We could draw strength from others, but we could not make comparisons.*
>
> **—AL BARRINEAU**
> **SUPPORT PARTNER**

Grade 2: Moderately differentiated tumors—About 25 - 50 percent of cells are abnormal. Between 50 - 75 percent of cells still resemble the parent cell. They are like first cousins. Term describes cells between the well and poorly differentiated stages.

Grade 3: Poorly differentiated cells—Nearly 50 - 75 percent of cells are abnormal; 25 - 50 percent of cells resemble the parent cell. Similar to third cousins. Usually aggressive.

Grade 4: Undifferentiated cells—More than 75 percent of the cells are abnormal. Only 25 percent or less of the cells in the tumor are normal. These cells do not resemble any family member. Usually most aggressive.

SCARFF/BLOOM/RICHARDSON TUMOR GRADING SCALE

Some pathologists use the Scarff/Bloom/Richardson grading scale. This grading system gives a number from 1 to 3 according to aggressiveness of three different characteristics of the tumor: tubular formation, nuclear size and shape, mitotic count. The numbers from each characteristic are then totaled to determine the aggressiveness of a tumor. The higher the number, the more aggressive the characteristics of the tumor.

1. Tubular Formation	Grade Value	Evaluates cell
Majority >75%	1	arrangement for
Moderate degree 10–75%	2	characteristics of looking
Little or none	3	like a small tube.
2. Nuclear Shape/Size	**Grade Value**	Evaluates size and
Uniform nuclear shapes	1	shape variation of cells
Moderate increase in varying shapes	2	and nucleus of cells.
Marked variation (often large nucleus)	3	
3. Cell Division Rate	**Grade Value**	Determines how many
Low (0–5)	1	cells are visible in the
Moderate degree (6–10)	2	dividing stage in an
High (>11)	3	area of the tumor.
Final Cumulative Total	**Points**	**Total of the scores in**
Grade 1 – well differentiated	3–5 points	**the above three areas**
Grade 2 – moderately differentiated	6–7 points	**of evaluation**
Grade 3 – poorly differentiated	8–9 points	**determines final grade.**

PROGNOSTIC TESTS

Various tests may be ordered to look at specific characteristics of the tumor cells. Some of these tests and markers may not be requested by your physician.

DNA Status: A test that looks at the genetic material found in the DNA (blueprint for cell reproduction) of a cell. Normal DNA of a cell appears with two sets of chromosomes.

DNA ploidy determines DNA composition of cells. Tumors may be diploid or aneuploid:

- Diploid means having two sets of chromosomes, which is normal.

- Aneuploid refers to the characteristic of having either fewer than or more than two sets of chromosomes; this is abnormal, suggesting a more aggressive form of cancer.

DNA index is the ratio of aneuploid DNA compared to diploid DNA.

PROLIFERATION MARKERS

- **S Phase Fraction**—Flow cytometry reveals number of dividing cells and corresponds to the growth rate of a tumor.

- **Mitotic Rate**—Microscopic observation of number of cells that are dividing.

- **Ki67 Stain**—Microscopic observation of all dividing cells.

Increase in any of the above proliferation markers suggests an aggressive tumor.

HORMONE RECEPTOR ASSAY

A hormone receptor assay is a chemical or observational test that measures the presence of estrogen and progesterone receptors in the tumor cells. It tells the physician whether the tumor was stimulated to grow by female hormones, and it is very important in determining what type of treatment will be used. If a tumor is positive, that means it was stimulated by estrogen or progesterone and usually carries a slight increase in a positive prognosis. Positive receptor tumors may be treated with anti-hormonal medications such as Tamoxifen for control.

Tumors may be:

- ER+ (positive) and PR+ (positive)
- ER- (negative) and PR+ (positive)
- ER+ (positive) and PR- (negative)
- ER- (negative) and PR- (negative)

HER-2/NEU ONCOGENE

HER-2/neu (c-erbB-2) oncogene is a substance in cells that promotes tumor development. This oncogene is found amplified and over-expressed in about 20-30% of breast cancers. Recently it has been demonstrated that HER-2/neu over-expression can predict the response to Adriamycin-based chemotherapy, as well as resistance to Tamoxifen. Furthermore, the recent introduction of immunotherapy with a "humanized" monoclonal antibody, Transmuxtab (Herceptin™) directed at the HER-2/neu protein, has required further screening of breast cancers for HER-2/neu over-expression to determine if these types of drugs may be effective.

There are many other diagnostic tests being used to evaluate tumors. Your physician will discuss the tests selected to evaluate your partner's tumor. Each of these tests helps to provide the pieces of the puzzle needed by the oncologist to determine the best treatment.

The pathologist prepares a written report that is sent to your physician. Times vary as to when the final report will be available. Check with your physician on how long the laboratory requires. After reviewing the pathology report, your physician will decide if further diagnostic tests, such as a bone scan, liver scan, chest x-ray, CT scan, or an MRI (magnetic resonance imaging) may be needed to stage her cancer.

When all the results are received from the tests, your partner's cancer will be staged on a scale from zero (in situ cancer) to four (a cancer with distant metastasis). A stage zero cancer is the earliest, and has the best prognosis. Staging is an estimate of how much the cancer has already spread and is important in selecting appropriate treatment.

BREAST CANCER STAGES

Three basic factors are considered in staging:

- tumor size
- lymph node involvement
- metastasis to other areas

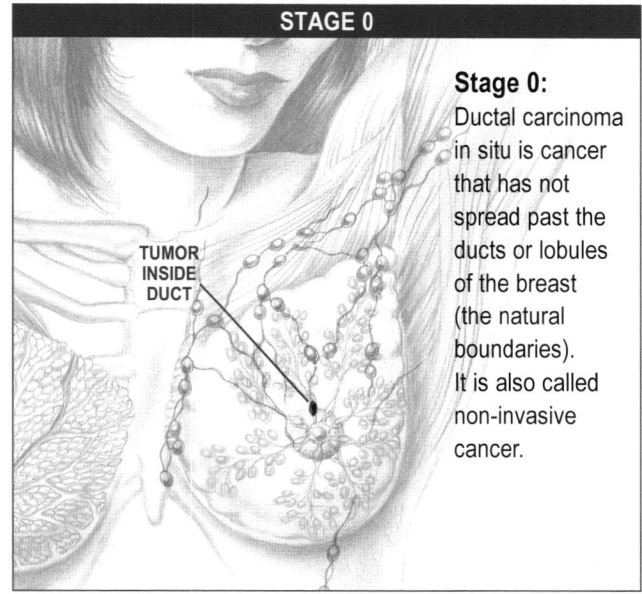

STAGE 0

TUMOR INSIDE DUCT

Stage 0: Ductal carcinoma in situ is cancer that has not spread past the ducts or lobules of the breast (the natural boundaries). It is also called non-invasive cancer.

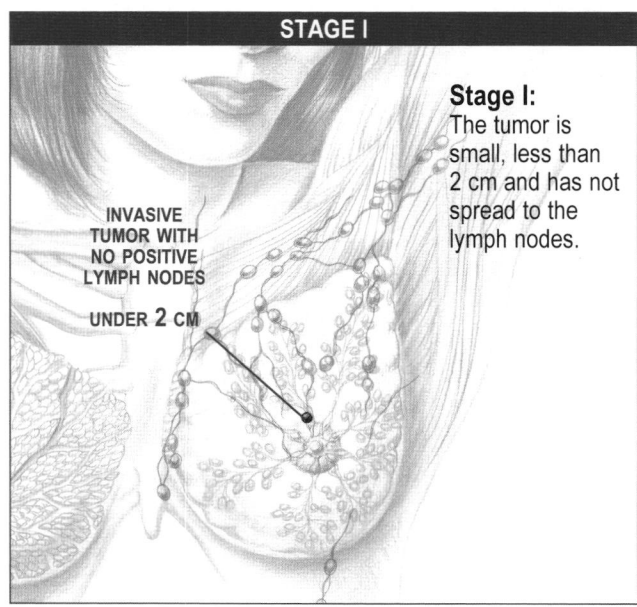

STAGE I

INVASIVE TUMOR WITH NO POSITIVE LYMPH NODES

UNDER 2 CM

Stage I: The tumor is small, less than 2 cm and has not spread to the lymph nodes.

STAGE II

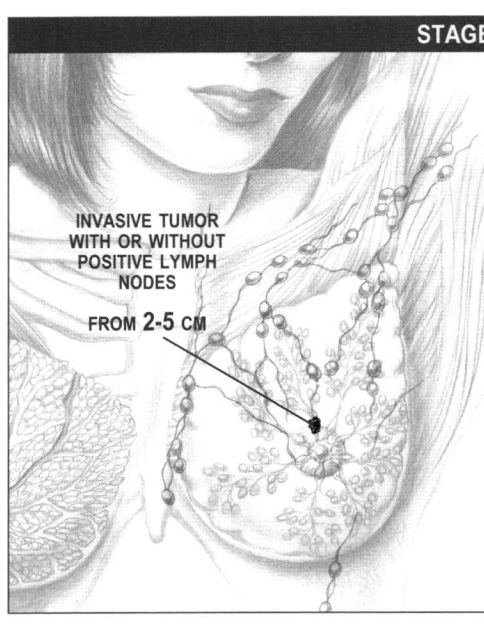

INVASIVE TUMOR WITH OR WITHOUT POSITIVE LYMPH NODES

FROM 2-5 CM

Stage II: Any one of these conditions:

- The tumor is less than 2 cm and has spread to the axillary lymph nodes under the arm

- The tumor is between 2 - 5 cm but has not spread to the axillary lymph nodes

- There is no evidence of a tumor in the breast, but there is cancer in the axillary lymph nodes

- The tumor is between 2 - 5 cm and has spread to the axillary lymph nodes

- The tumor is larger than 5 cm but has not spread to the axillary lymph nodes

STAGE III

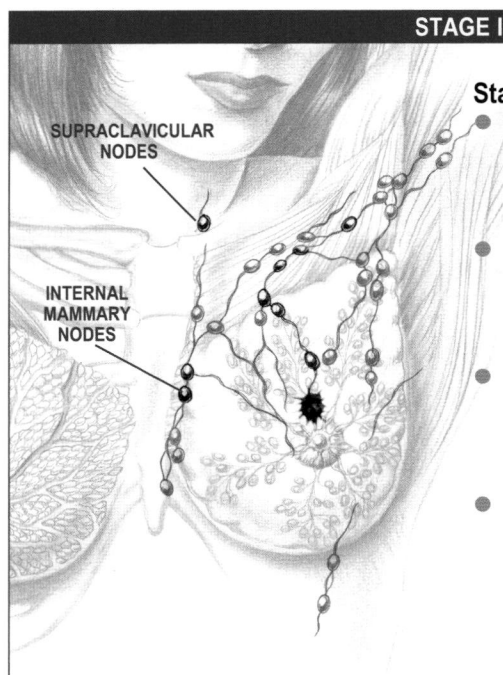

SUPRACLAVICULAR NODES

INTERNAL MAMMARY NODES

Stage III: Any of these conditions:

- The tumor is smaller than 5 cm and has spread to the axillary lymph nodes that are attached to each other or to other structures

- The tumor is larger than 5 cm and has spread to the axillary lymph nodes, which may or may not be attached to each other or to other structures

- The tumor has spread to the chest wall or caused swelling or ulceration of the breast or is diagnosed as inflammatory breast cancer.

- A tumor of any size that has not spread to distant parts of the body, but has spread to the lymph nodes above the collarbone, under the collarbone, or both the nodes inside the breast and the internal mammary nodes.

STAGE IV

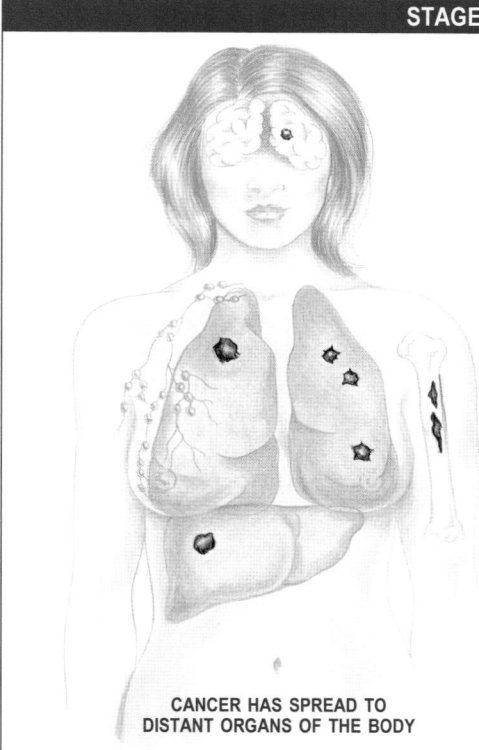

CANCER HAS SPREAD TO
DISTANT ORGANS OF THE BODY

Stage IV: Distant Metastasis

The tumor can be any size and has spread to other sites in the body, usually the bones, lung, liver or brain.

NOTE:
Recurrent Breast Cancer

Breast cancer is called recurrent if the cancer has come back (recurred) after it was first diagnosed and treated. Recurrent breast cancer may occur at any stage. It may come back in the breast (called a local recurrence), in the chest wall, or in another part of the body like in distant organs, bones or other lymph nodes (also called distant metastasis), stage IV.

When your partner returns to the physician for her pathology results, she may want to ask the following questions and write down the answers. Some doctors will provide a copy of the pathology report for her records, and some pathologists will discuss the report with the patient.

105

REMEMBER

THE PATHOLOGY REPORT
CONTAINS INFORMATION
NEEDED TO DETERMINE
TREATMENT DECISIONS.

INDIVIDUALS MUST DECIDE
HOW MUCH THEY WISH
TO UNDERSTAND ABOUT
THEIR CANCER.

AS A SUPPORT PARTNER,
IT IS MOST
HELPFUL IF YOU ASSIST
HER IN GETTING
THE PATHOLOGY REPORT
AND UNDERSTANDING IT
TO THE DEGREE THAT SHE
FEELS COMFORTABLE.

QUESTIONS TO ASK ABOUT THE PATHOLOGY REPORT:

- What is the name of the type of cancer?

- Was the tumor in situ (inside ducts) or infiltrating (invasive, grown through the cell walls)?

- What size was the tumor? (The size is in centimeters or millimeters.)

- Was the cancer found anywhere else in the breast tissue? (The term multifocal means additional cancer was found in the same quadrant as the tumor; multicentric means it was found in another quadrant of the breast distant from the tumor.)

- How many lymph nodes were removed?

- For sentinel node surgery: How many sentinel nodes were removed?

- Were any lymph nodes positive with cancer cells?

- Were the tumor receptors estrogen or progesterone positive or negative?

- Was the tumor HER-2/neu positive or negative?

- Was the cancer diploid (like a normal, original cell) or aneuploid (unlike normal cells)?

- What was the S phase, mitotic index or proliferative status (how fast cancer is/was growing at time of surgery).

- Is there anything else we need to know about her cancer?

TREATMENTS FOR BREAST CANCER

After the final pathology report is studied, the oncologist (a physician who treats cancer) will recommend a plan of treatment. This may include chemotherapy (treatment with cancer-fighting drugs), radiation therapy (x-ray), or hormonal therapy. Medical oncologists specialize in treating patients with chemotherapy and radiation oncologists specialize in radiation therapy. Some women will receive all of these treatment methods. Others may only receive one type of treatment. Some may not receive any treatment because of their tumor characteristics and the surgery performed.

Oncologists carefully review the pathology report and any other tests, perform a thorough physical exam, and then prescribe a treatment plan.

This treatment plan is designed according to:

- cancer cell type
- size of tumor
- in situ or invasive cancer
- growth rate of tumor
- tumor markers (HER-2)
- evidence of spread of cancer
- lymph node involvement
- how much the cells have changed from original cells
- estrogen and progesterone hormone receptor status
- menopausal state of the patient
- medical history and general health

> " *As a little league football coach, I learned that the first step to winning is to build a good team. I thought about this when my mate faced a breast cancer diagnosis. If we were to win this game, we needed the best team. Our family doctor acted as head coach, my wife became the quarterback, and, at times, I only felt like the water boy; but, by putting together the best medical and supportive team we could, we knew we were doing all that was humanly possible to give her the best chance for recovery.* "
>
> **—AL BARRINEAU**
> **SUPPORT PARTNER**

Remember, there is more than one kind of breast cancer, and different types of cancers may require different treatment. Some types of cancer, and cancer that has spread to other parts of the body, may require chemotherapy administration before surgery is performed. Do not compare your partner's treatment with another patient's treatment because you will probably be comparing two entirely different cases.

CHEMOTHERAPY

Chemotherapy drugs are usually given intravenously (through a vein), but occasionally they are administered by pill. Treatments usually consist of a combination of several drugs. They begin several weeks past final surgery and are given in a clinic or a physician's office. Frequency of administration varies according to the treatment plan and is usually completed in four to six months. Side effects vary according to the drugs, amount of drugs administered, and the individual patient. The treatment team will supply information on the drugs and on management of side effects.

Some women with poor veins (hard to find with an IV needle), or those who are to receive certain types of drugs may require a permanent device inserted under the skin called a venous access device or a "port" ("port-a-cath"). This device is usually placed under the skin on the chest wall during a brief outpatient surgery and is used to administer chemotherapy and draw blood samples. The patient is able to perform normal activities with the device, including bathing and swimming.

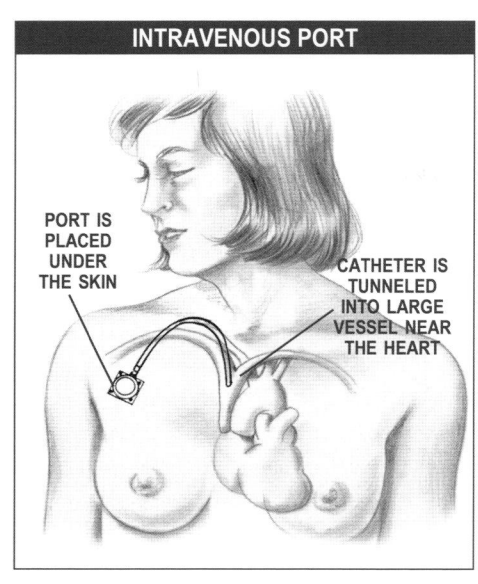

INTRAVENOUS PORT

PORT IS PLACED UNDER THE SKIN

CATHETER IS TUNNELED INTO LARGE VESSEL NEAR THE HEART

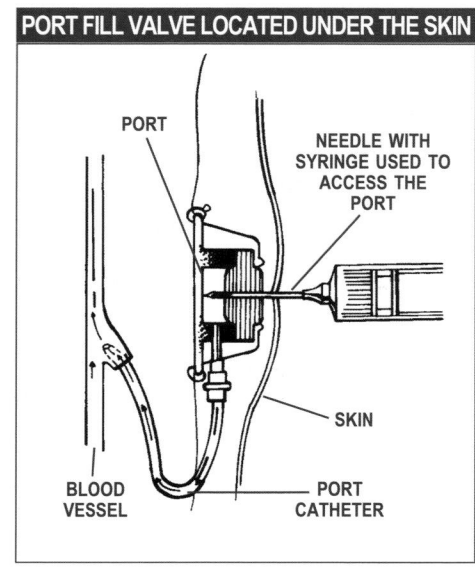

PORT FILL VALVE LOCATED UNDER THE SKIN

PORT

NEEDLE WITH SYRINGE USED TO ACCESS THE PORT

SKIN

BLOOD VESSEL

PORT CATHETER

RADIATION THERAPY

Radiation therapy is used after a lumpectomy or for local control when cancer has spread into an area. The breast area is radiated by a machine that produces high energy x-rays from radioactive substances to kill any remaining cancer cells in the area.

Treatment usually begins when the incision has healed—usually after four to six weeks—or it may be started at the completion of chemotherapy treatments. On the initial visit the area is carefully marked for future treatment. Thereafter, each treatment only takes minutes to deliver, with the appointment time allowing extra time to undress and have a technologist check your records and set the adjustments on the machine. Treatments are given on a daily basis, Monday through Friday, ranging from five to seven weeks. Side effects are generally mild but may include changes in the skin over the treated area similar to a mild sunburn, mild fatigue, and, occasionally, a sore throat. The treatment team will provide information on the management of side effects.

HORMONAL THERAPY

Hormonal therapy may be recommended if the studies performed on the tumor prove to be positive for stimulation by estrogen (ER+) or progesterone (PR+). There are four major kinds of hormonal therapy. The decision of the appropriate drug will be based, in part, on whether a woman is pre or post menopausal. Some of the drugs lower the amount of estrogen in the body, some block estrogen receptors on the cells and some shut down the production of estrogen in the body.

Drug Categories:

- **Aromatase inhibitors** reduce the amount of estrogen the body produces in post-menopausal women. Three of the drugs are Arimidex (anastrozole), Aromasin (exemestane) and Femra (letrozole).
- **SERMS (Selective Estrogen-Receptor Modulators)** block the estrogen receptors on the cell so that estrogen cannot enter. The two drugs used are Nolvadex (tamoxifen) and Evista (raloxifene).
- **ERDs (estrogen-receptor down regulators)** destroy the estrogen receptor on the cell. The drug currently in use is Faslocex (fulvestrant).
- **Ovarian shutdown** or removal drugs are Zoladex (groserelin) and Lupron (leuprolide), and they are given by injection once a month for several months.

Hormonal medication may be given in many different ways: alone, in combination or one after the other.

BREAST CANCER GENETIC TESTING

In 1994 and 1995, two mutated (changed) genes, BRCA1 and BRCA2 (BR=breast, CA=cancer), were discovered that cause 7 – 10 percent of breast cancers. A blood test can now determine if a person is a carrier of either of these mutated genes and the possible cause of her breast cancer. These two genes also cause a woman to be at high risk for ovarian cancer.

After a breast cancer diagnosis, the healthcare team can review the patient's family and personal history to determine if she meets the criteria for genetic testing. One important factor about genetic mutations is that they can be inherited from a mother or father. Breast or ovarian cancer in the history of either parent is an important consideration. For years, only the mother's family history was considered to put a woman at higher risk. We now know that the risk comes equally from the father.

Genetic testing can determine if she has a mutation in either of these identified genes. If positive, her children, male or female, are at a 50 percent risk of inheriting these defective genes, which they can then pass on to their offspring. Having a mutated gene places them at higher risk for breast, ovarian, or other cancers.

Estimated Lifetime Risk

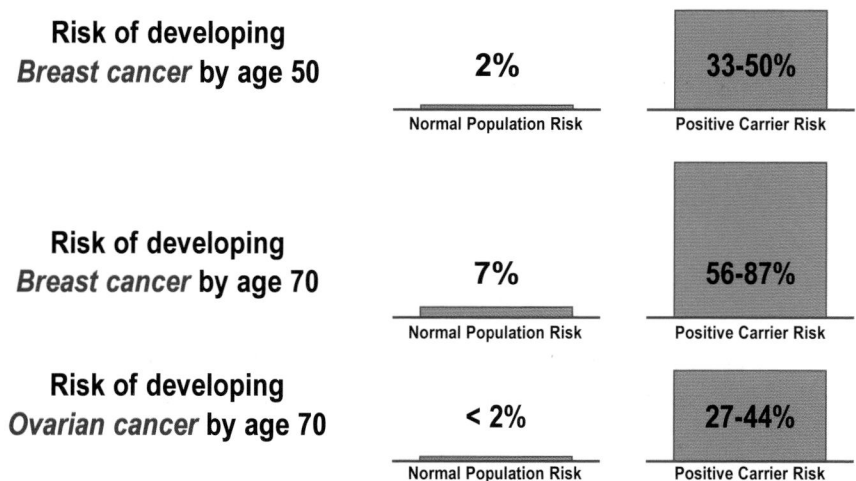

Risk of developing
Breast cancer **by age 50**   **2%**   **33-50%**

Normal Population Risk   Positive Carrier Risk

Risk of developing
Breast cancer **by age 70**   **7%**   **56-87%**

Normal Population Risk   Positive Carrier Risk

Risk of developing
Ovarian cancer **by age 70**   **< 2%**   **27-44%**

Normal Population Risk   Positive Carrier Risk

COURTESY OF MYRIAD GENETICS

Criteria for BRCA1 or BRCA2 Testing:

- Individuals with a personal or family history of breast cancer before age 50 or ovarian cancer at any age
- Individuals with two or more primary diagnoses of breast and/or ovarian cancer
- Individuals of Ashkenazi Jewish descent with a personal or family history of breast cancer before age of 50 or ovarian cancer at any age
- Male breast cancer patients

Benefits of Testing

- Allows one to know if their cancer was related to one of these mutated genes
- A negative test, showing no gene mutation, means that the gene for breast cancer was not passed on to children of the patient. Prevents unnecessary anxiety about children being high risk and prevents future expensive surveillance tests.
- Positive test allows family members to choose to be tested or placed in high risk surveillance programs
- Positive test may also alter recommendations for future treatment of breast cancer and indicate a need for surveillance for ovarian cancer or prophylactic surgical removal of ovaries

If your partner has a history of breast cancer or ovarian cancer on either side of the family, discuss with a qualified healthcare provider the benefits from genetic testing. Testing consists of having a vial or syringe (several tablespoons) of blood drawn and sent to a laboratory for testing. It is suggested that the patient be counseled about the procedure before blood is drawn and tested and after the test results are given.

For up-to-date information on genetic breast cancer visit the Web site www.myriadtests.com.

CLINICAL TRIALS

Occasionally, as part of treatment decisions, some women may have the opportunity to participate in new treatments called clinical trials. These are new investigational studies that research the planning of highly effective treatment and prevention strategies. Thousands of research studies are currently under way in the United States. Most trials are conducted by the National Cancer Institute, major medical centers, or pharmaceutical companies. If a new treatment is determined safe and effective at the completion of the trial, the U.S. Food and Drug Administration (FDA) grants approval for their widespread commercial use by patients.

Four Phases of Clinical Trials:

- Phase I trials are designed to find out if a promising new therapy is worthy of further investigation.

- Phase II trials confirm the value of the drug and determine the dosage and administration of the drug.

- Phase III is the final phase and requires a large number of patients to receive either the standard therapy or the newer therapy in order to compare beneficial survival results and quality of life during treatment. If one drug is found to be more effective than the standard one, the trial is stopped and all participants are eligible for the more successful treatment. If there is any evidence that the newer drug is inferior or has unusually toxic side effects, the experimental medication is discontinued.

- Phase IV trials are done to make sure results of Phase III are applicable to the general patient population.

Clinical Trial Informed Consent

Your doctor or nurse will explain in detail the type and purpose of the trial. The patient will be given an informed consent form to read and sign. This form must include the expected benefits, the negative aspects, other treatment options, assurance that your personal records will be kept confidential, the negatives aspects, and a statement indicating that your participation is voluntary and you may withdraw at any time.

Participating in the trial does not prevent you from getting any additional medical care you may need. If you decide to participate in the trial, you will need to contact your insurance provider to ask if it covers any charges. Be sure the researchers are aware if your plan does not cover the costs of clinical trials. Some trials are simply a comparison of two drugs or timing of administration to determine which is more effective. Your physician will explain the details of the trial.

Questions To Ask About Clinical Trials

- What phase is the clinical trial in that you recommend? (Phase I, II, III or IV)

- Who is sponsoring the study? (Needs to be approved by a reputable national group like the National Cancer Institute, a major teaching institution, or the FDA.)

- What is the purpose of this study?

- What advantage does this trial have compared to standard recommended treatment?

- How long will the clinical trial last?

- Where will treatments be given and evaluated while on the trial?

- Is the drug/combination of drugs available outside the clinical trial? (Some drugs may be available to your physician outside the clinical trial.)

- How will the success of the treatment be evaluated? (blood tests, scans, etc.)

- How much additional time will participating in the trial require over standard treatment?

- Will there be any extra expenses or will all costs of the trial be covered?

- Will our insurance company cover the cost of the trial?

- What type of follow-up will continue after the trial is completed?

Understanding Clinical Trials

If you want to know more about clinical trials, the most obvious place to start is with your oncologist. The Cancer Information Service (CIS), a program supported by the National Cancer Institute, can compile information about the latest nationwide cancer treatments for a specific type and stage of cancer. For more information on clinical trials you can access the Physician's Data Query (PDQ) at www.cancertrials.nci.nih.gov.

Patient advocacy groups such as the National Alliance of Breast Cancer Organizations (NABCO) at 1-888-80-NABCO and the American Cancer Society (ACS) at 1-800-ACS-2345 also have patient information on participating in clinical trials and other relevant information on new trials.

To Participate or Not To Participate

The decision is often not an easy one to make. This decision is very personal, and one that can only be made after the patient has discussed the advantages and disadvantages with her physician and clinical trials nurse. You can best help by assisting her in getting her questions answered about participating in the trial. When the final decision is made, she needs to feel that she has chosen what is best for her. Some women prefer the "tried and known" while others feel that they are getting an even better chance by taking a newer drug or drug combination. Some feel that by their participation in clinical trials they will be helping other women in the future. Remember, no one has the right answer to the question of whether or not one should or should not participate; there is not an absolute answer. That is why it is called a "trial."

REMEMBER

TREATMENT IS BASED ON THE FINAL SURGICAL PATHOLOGY REPORT AND THE INDIVIDUAL CHARACTER-ISTICS OF THE PATIENT TO DETERMINE THE NEED FOR CHEMOTHERAPY, RADIATION THERAPY, OR HORMONAL THERAPY.

BRCA1 AND BRCA2 GENES ARE INHERITED GENES THAT PLACE A WOMAN AT EXTREMELY HIGH RISK FOR BREAST OR OVARIAN CANCER. TESTING CAN IDENTIFY THOSE WHO CARRY THE GENE.

CLINICAL TRIALS ARE STUDIES TO DETERMINE MORE EFFECTIVE METHODS TO TREAT DISEASE. WHETHER OR NOT TO PARTICIPATE IN A CLINICAL TRIAL IS A CHOICE SOME WOMEN MAY BE ASKED TO MAKE.

FOCUS GROUP DATA

EduCare Inc. conducted research during 2000 and 2001 on sexuality after breast cancer treatment in focus groups of breast cancer survivors. The groups were convened in 11 different hospitals nationally. The purpose of the groups was to gather information from women who had taken chemotherapy on the impact it had on their sexual functioning and quality of life. Investigated were the physical changes experienced, the sexual changes, the impact on the relationship with their sexual partner, their educational needs before treatment, and the women's request for future services of pre-treatment education and support to be offered by their healthcare team and facility.

Judy C. Kneece, RN, OCN conducted the focus groups, with patients invited from their health-care facility who hosted the groups. Groups were held in the southeast, northeast, midwest and southwest. A total of 126 survivors responded to 143 questions using individual Audience Response Interactive data pads. These hand-held computer pads allowed all answers to be anonymous. Each woman was free to express her true feelings without anyone knowing how she answered. The computer automatically analyzed the data entered at each individual site and then combined the 11 sites for the final analysis. Included throughout this book are portions of the data gathered.

YOUR PARTNERSHIP IN RECOVERY

The chronic phase of recovery for the patient, partner, and family begins when the patient returns home. The acute emotions of the diagnosis slip into the background while the conflict of merging new family roles with the old routines—meals, cleaning, laundry, jobs, school—becomes the focus. The patient often struggles with the realization that she may not be able to physically maintain her role in the family immediately after surgery or during some chemotherapy treatments. Change becomes difficult as your family life takes on a lower emotional tone and you concentrate on reassigning the chores of daily living. As a mate, you will strengthen your family relationship by becoming a part of the solution to the routine chores.

Look for opportunities to help in her physical as well as emotional recovery. When your partner returns home, she will probably need to have her dressing changed and her drain bulbs emptied. Some women appreciate assistance, while others feel uncomfortable. Ask her how you and the family can be more helpful. The surgeon will instruct your partner on when to begin an exercise program that will help her regain strength and mobility in her surgical arm. One patient's support partner became the "captain of her physical therapy team." The partner reminded her of her exercises and helped her perform them. By participating with her in the dull, routine exercise series, this partner restored a vital sense of caring in the patient's mind. This teamwork kept them emotionally in touch during a time of physical readjustment for both of them.

> *The one I loved most was battling for her life. We were in this together.*
>
> —AL BARRINEAU
> SUPPORT PARTNER

SUPPORT DURING TREATMENTS

Chemotherapy or radiation treatments may be required after surgery (see Chapter 15 on chemotherapy). The time of treatments can be very anxiety-provoking for your partner. While she will probably be physically able to go for her treatments alone, psychologically she may need someone to accompany her, especially on the first visits. A support person—you, a family member, or friend—can help relieve her anxiety and help her understand the oncologist's explanations about her treatments. Your mate may be hesitant to ask for you to go with her, but she will

> *I do not like hospitals. I do not like being around sick people. But the person I loved most in the world was having to have chemotherapy treatments in our fight to save her life. I was glad to go with her.*
>
> **—AL BARRINEAU**
> **SUPPORT PARTNER**

be very grateful when you offer to go or find someone else to accompany her. Others may not want "so much fuss" made over their treatments and will feel more in control if they go alone when they are physically able. Communicating your willingness and desire to share this time is important to her.

Planning to be helpful during treatments begins by understanding what her treatments involve. Your oncologist and staff will answer the following questions to help you and your partner plan and adjust during chemotherapy and/or radiation treatments:

- How often will treatments be administered?
- How long will each treatment session last?
- Is someone allowed to be with the patient during these treatments?
- What are the expected side effects of the treatment and when do they occur?
- Will any medication be given prior to or after treatments that could prevent her from driving?
- At what time during the treatment cycle will she become the most fatigued?
- At what time during the treatment cycle will she be most vulnerable to infections?
- Are there any side effects, signs, or symptoms that need to be recognized and reported to the healthcare team?

By understanding these facts you will be able to make this time as psychologically and physically comfortable as possible. Plan to have food available around treatment dates so she will not feel responsible for meals. She may wish to schedule treatments to be given on

Fridays, so you may take over household responsibilities on the weekend, allowing her plenty of time to rest. One couple made a ritual of renting several movies and made this their weekend to catch up on their movie watching. The children pulled their sleeping bags into the den, and everyone "camped out" around Mom. The weekend was eagerly anticipated instead of dreaded, despite the physical discomfort experienced by the patient. Carefully assess her physical and psychological needs so you may be as supportive as possible during treatment.

Treatments may physically drain and fatigue the patient, resulting in her inability to resume her prior lifestyle and routines. Her daily responsibilities may have to be redistributed among family members, co-workers, and friends. One husband told of his experience taking on unaccustomed chores. "I already did most of the cooking, but I learned to do the laundry, only ruining a few items as I learned. I must confess, I found out what caused pink underwear. We had a cleaning person come in one day a week on a regular basis. The expense was not too great and was certainly worth the energy it saved. Ideally, I wanted the kids to do more; however, they are normal and haven't become much more useful around the house." Recognize the need for changes in household chores, family, work, and community activities. Take the initiative in reassigning responsibilities and helping your mate prioritize her duties during recovery.

UNDERSTANDING THE SIDE EFFECTS OF CHEMOTHERAPY ON THE RELATIONSHIP
Chemotherapy treatments may impact a relationship both physically and mentally. You will receive much information on how to manage physical side effects such as nausea, diarrhea, low white blood cell counts, and the resulting fatigue. Your oncologist will provide medications and helpful interventions to control these side effects. However, several other side effects—fatigue, hair loss, and sexuality changes—may profoundly impact your relationship, requiring special understanding and support from you.

HAIR LOSS–
THE MOST PAINFUL SIDE EFFECT
Many women have expressed that the loss of their hair through chemotherapy treatments was the most distressing of all losses during breast cancer. Even though the loss is temporary, and the hair returns after treatment is completed, women have described its impact as "being more upsetting than the loss of my breast." Hair loss is difficult because it is outward evidence of the cancer process. It is often the first visible public

> *When my wife lost her hair during chemotherapy treatments, it was almost the proverbial 'straw that broke the camel's back.' Losing her hair seemed to strip her of the last defense she had in denial of her own cancer.*
>
> **—AL BARRINEAU**
> **SUPPORT PARTNER**

display of their battles with cancer. It is much easier to camouflage the loss or alteration of a breast under clothing than the loss of hair with a wig.

The amount and timing of hair loss will vary according to the kind of drugs, the dosage of the drugs and the individual response to the drugs given. Most hair loss occurs between two and four weeks after the first treatment. Some treatment regimens will only cause gradual hair thinning; others will cause complete hair loss. To help you and your partner prepare for this occurrence in the treatment process, discuss with the treatment team how much hair loss to expect and when it may occur.

To help your partner deal with her hair loss, discuss what you have learned and assure her of your total acceptance. It is recommended that she shop for a wig before she loses her hair to better match her hair color and style. Her wig will probably not be noticeable except to those who know she has lost her hair. Do not complain about the cost of wigs or insist on her getting one that she does not feel comfortable wearing. She needs your support and understanding during this extremely sensitive time.

ALOPECIA

When women in a focus group who had complete hair loss (alopecia) were asked to rate their emotional reactions to losing their hair:

- 50% reported it as severely emotionally painful

- 42% as moderately emotionally painful

- only 8% of no emotional consequence

When participants were asked to distinguish which was more emotionally distressing, their altered body image change from surgery or hair loss, 74% reported hair loss as being the most emotionally painful.

Those experiencing complete hair loss were asked if they allowed their sexual partner to see them with their heads uncovered. 90% reported yes and 10% reported keeping their heads covered at all times.

Women were asked to rate on a scale of 1 to 10 the impact that alopecia had on their sexual functioning. The overall score was 4.8, or a moderate impact.

Obviously, the day or week she loses her hair will be one of her lowest emotional times. You can't change it. You can't make things different. Your best response is your reassuring presence. Allow her to grieve her loss and shed her tears as she feels is necessary.

Many people revert to jokes and humor during uncomfortable and painful times. However, support partners advise against using nicknames such as "Baldie," "Kojak," or other terms denoting hair loss. She may laugh outwardly but may inwardly feel different. Let her take the lead in how she can best react and manage her new appearance. Respect her privacy as she dresses and undresses. For some women, it may be more difficult to allow you to see her bald head than to let you see her scar. Remember, hair loss is usually temporary. Therefore, don't insist that she show you her bald head or thinning hair if she feels uncomfortable. This will pass, unlike the change in her body image.

Some women will cling to the security of their wigs after their hair begins to return. She may need your encouragement to shed the wig and show off her new, shorter haircut. For some, this takes courage because they may have entered treatment with longer hair and may only feel comfortable returning to that image. This can be especially difficult if they feel that longer hair was important to you. Let her know of your acceptance early in the treatment phase.

> *I wanted Anna to know that I, too, felt the emotional pain of her having to undergo treatment. When she had her first chemo treatment, I shaved my head, hoping in some way this would comfort her. I don't necessarily recommend this for others, but it helped me show her what I couldn't say.*
>
> *I tried to make getting better the only thing she had to worry about during her treatment. This was one thing I could "fix" for her.*
>
> —BRIAN CLUXTON
> SUPPORT PARTNER

BIRTH CONTROL DURING TREATMENT

Birth control should be discussed with the physician if your partner is premenopausal. Since there is no way to accurately predict if a woman will continue to ovulate and have menstrual periods, birth control is recommended. Chemotherapy drugs could cause birth defects if pregnancy should occur. Birth control pills are not recommended because of their hormonal composition. Spermicidal agents or barrier methods such as condoms or diaphragms are recommended. A decision made by some couples, who have completed their families, is tubal ligation, a minor surgical procedure where a woman's fallopian tubes are cut. This is often done at the time of breast surgery to prevent having to return for a second procedure and additional sedation. Some couples choose that their male partner have a vasectomy.

WEIGHT GAIN AFTER TREATMENT

Many women gain weight during and after breast cancer treatment. Reasons given by medical clinicians include decreased activity with increased caloric intake, fluid retention from drugs, and effects on body metabolism from anti-hormonal drugs. Most women report that it was as if their metabolism changed overnight after treatment. Even with the same amount of calories as before, they gained weight. Even with an increase in physical activity after the treatment their weight did not drop to pretreatment levels.

Weight gain is another potential obstacle for some women regarding their self-esteem that can affect sexual functioning. As you can tell from the focus group, 89 percent of women said it had an impact on sexual self-perception. As a supportive partner, understanding that weight gain is not necessarily a lack of self-control but a change of normal body metabolism will lay the foundation for acceptance. We live in a culture where we are constantly told that a slim body is the desired norm for sexual attractiveness. For many women, this is a very difficult change to deal with. Expressing your understanding, if she does gain weight, is a way to remove an obstacle for future sexual functioning.

WEIGHT GAIN

54% of the participants reported gaining weight during or after treatment.

Those that gained weight were asked if they felt it affected their self-image and eventually had an effect on their sexual relationships.

An overwhelming 53% answered yes, 36% said that it had some impact and 11% said it had no impact.

One way to help is to encourage her to get regular physical exercise. Suggest a regular activity together or as a family (not so that she will lose weight, or you may lose your influence) to have a regular time to share with each other. Activities such as a walking program, swimming, golfing, bowling, dancing, aerobic exercise classes, hiking, yoga classes, or Pilates classes (stretching and muscle strength building exercises) as a couple can strengthen a relationship. These are healthy and stress reducing activities and may cause both of your waistlines to decrease. However, the major focus should always be good health, not her weight.

INSOMNIA

Most women have problems sleeping all night starting from the time they find an abnormality in their breast, throughout treatment, and well into recovery. Insomnia can be a continuing problem for women who take chemotherapy and remain in a menopausal condition.

INSOMNIA

Data from the focus groups indicated that 88% of the women experienced insomnia during treatment, 70% six months after treatment, and 60% still suffered a year after treatment ended.

The inability to sleep all night can contribute to fatigue, irritability, mental fogginess, and depression. This often becomes like the chicken and egg debate: which comes first—these symptoms or insomnia? The appropriate answer is that whatever the cause, insomnia should be addressed and interventions offered by a healthcare provider. It should not be experienced week after week and dismissed as normal and not important enough to ask for help. Chronic insomnia needs treatment; a night or two of interrupted sleep can be tolerated, but continued insomnia can cause grave coping and quality of life problems.

STRESS

Stress is expected during a cancer diagnosis. During interviews with women in the focus groups experiencing insomnia, the severity of sleeplessness correlated closely with the level of stress they were under (highest during diagnostic and early treatment phase). For women who are regularly not sleeping all night because of stress, medications can greatly reduce insomnia. Sleeping medications are recommended for short-term use and are appropriate for a limited time. However, many women complain of continued drowsiness the next day and find that other options offer nearer to normal functioning the next day. Anti-anxiety medications can relieve stress and allow women to sleep. Benadryl, an over-the-counter antihistamine is a safe sedative for most people. Encourage her to contact her healthcare provider for medications to help with her anxiety and lack of sleep.

For women who take chemotherapy, insomnia may be increased significantly in relation to the number of hot flashes and night sweats experienced by the patient. For these women, asking their healthcare provider for interventions to reduce hot flashes and night sweats is essential. One woman in the focus group had not slept longer than 2 – 3 hours a night since treatment that had ended two years earlier because of hot flashes. This is unacceptable. Hot flashes or night sweats that cause waking deserve attention.

HOT FLASHES

Hot flashes can be reduced greatly for most women by taking an SSRI (Selective Serotonin Reuptake Inhibitors) such as Celexa, Paxil, Prozac, Zoloft, Lexapro or Luvox. These drugs also assist with reducing depression and insomnia. For hot flashes or night sweats that do not respond to these interventions, a blood pressure medication, Clonidine (Catapres), has proven helpful for many women suffering severe symptoms. A combination of medications can reduce symptoms of insomnia, hot flashes, and night sweats to a manageable level. It is important to consider quality of life issues and to understand that they need and deserve attention from her healthcare provider. This may mean changing providers to find one that addresses all issues, and not just her cancer.

FOCUS GROUP DATA - HOT FLASHES

Hot Flashes	None	1-2 a Day	3-5 a Day	6-10 a Day	Over 10 a Day
Before Diagnosis	81%	10%	8%	0%	0%
During Treatment	32%	19%	25%	11%	13%
6 Months After Treatment	12%	26%	32%	13%	17%
12 Months After Treatment	14%	25%	27%	20%	14%

FOCUS GROUP DATA - NIGHT SWEATS

Night Sweats	None	1-2 a Day	3-5 a Day	6-10 a Day	Over 10 a Day
Before Diagnosis	75%	22%	3%	0%	0%
During Treatment	33%	25%	29%	9%	6%
6 Months After Treatment	25%	28%	36%	7%	4%
12 Months After Treatment	26%	42%	17%	9%	5%

REMEMBER

CHANGES IN SEXUAL FUNCTIONING CAN BE CAUSED BY SIDE EFFECTS OF TREATMENT.

HAIR LOSS CAN BE THE MOST TRAUMATIC OF ALL EVENTS FOR A BREAST CANCER PATIENT.

BIRTH CONTROL SHOULD BE DISCUSSED WITH THE PHYSICIAN AND BE USED
BEFORE AND AFTER TREATMENT IF A WOMAN IS PREMENOPAUSAL

WEIGHT GAIN CAN IMPACT SEXUAL SELF-PERCEPTION.
YOUR RESPONSE CAN PREVENT THIS FROM BEING AN OBSTACLE TO YOUR
SEXUAL RELATIONSHIP BY VERBALIZING ACCEPTANCE.

CHRONIC INSOMNIA, NIGHT SWEATS AND HOT FLASHES
CAN SERIOUSLY IMPAIR QUALITY OF LIFE
AND COPING CAPABILITIES.

SEXUALITY AFTER BREAST CANCER

"After treatment, my husband felt very rejected because I had no desire for sex and was unable to respond to him sexually. This caused a lot of stress and negative feelings for three years. I kept asking my doctors for help for years, but to no avail. My husband and I finally sat down and discussed everything. I then went to a new OB/GYN and once again asked for help. Thank goodness, she helped us solve our problem with various interventions. Today we have a very good sexual relationship. But we missed out on at least three years due to lack of knowledge about what we could do. I don't believe either of us would have opted to skip chemo just for me to be sexually responsive. But it would have been very helpful to know what to expect before chemo and then to get help dealing with the side effects without having to wait 3 years."

— EduCare Focus Group Participant

Sexuality issues after breast cancer are the least discussed of all breast cancer issues. In a national study of 126 women who had breast cancer surgery followed by chemotherapy, only 13 percent had any type of pretreatment discussion with anyone on their healthcare team about the potential effects from chemotherapy. This left an overwhelming 87 percent who were not forewarned of the potential for sexual dysfunction from chemotherapy treatments. After treatment started, an additional 5 percent had a

> *Sex was a difficult subject for me. I didn't want to make sexual advances, nor did I want Anna to think that she was not still as beautiful, sexy, and desirable to me as before. I didn't want to put any pressure on her. I finally expressed my reservations and we talked through the issues. This helped both of us greatly.*
>
> **—BRIAN CLUXTON**
> **SUPPORT PARTNER**

123

healthcare provider discuss sexual issues. In this group, 82 percent of women and their sexual partners were left to discover the changes that would occur from treatment themselves and to find their own ways to deal with them.

SEXUAL EDUCATION

- Of the 18% of women who had discussions with healthcare providers about sexuality issues, the average length of time ranged from 2 – 4 minutes, revealing how little emphasis is placed on sexuality. When these women rated their discussion value on a scale of 1 (not helpful) to 10 (very helpful) they rated the value of the discussion at 6.4 or of moderate help to the issues they faced.

- When asked if they questioned a physician/nurse about their sexual functioning during treatment, 32% responded yes. However, 100% reported having questions or problems. Those that asked questions rated the information provided by their healthcare providers a 4.1, slightly less than somewhat helpful. When asked if a suggested intervention was effective, the respondents rated the helpfulness of the intervention recommended by a physician/nurse a mere 3.9.

- Participants were asked, "How important do you think it is for a physician or nurse to discuss and offer suggestions about potential sexuality changes?" On a scale of 1 to 10, the group rated the need at a whopping 9.4. When asked about the need for healthcare providers giving written information about dealing with sexuality changes, they rated the need for written information at 9.4.

- In response to the question, "Would you have found it helpful for the physician/nurse to have included your partner in this sexuality discussion?" The response received an 8.9 rating on a scale from 1 to 10. Further clarification of this response came when the participants were asked, "Did you feel that your partner understood the multitude of changes you were experiencing during treatment that impacted your sexuality?" The question received a 5.3 rating, indicating the partner only somewhat understood.

The purpose of this chapter is to help you understand as a support partner the impact of chemotherapy on sexual functioning. It will also offer suggestions about what you need to know to help your partner adjust and prevent sexuality issues from becoming a roadblock to complete recovery. Focus group attendees (89 percent) wanted their partners to understand what they were facing by having the discussion with their healthcare provider. They often expressed that they did not understand it themselves and found it difficult to explain to their partner. About half of them reported (53 percent) that they felt their partners did not fully understand. Our goal is to help reduce problems in your relationship from lack of understanding.

COMMUNICATION ABOUT SEXUALITY

The first and major recommendation for sexual adjustment after breast cancer is open communication between you and your partner and your healthcare team. This is where problem solving begins, and it should begin early. With information you can anticipate changes and be prepared to deal with them emotionally and physically.

Often, when patients complain to their healthcare provider about sexuality issues, their complaints are taken lightly, which may cause the patient to think that sexuality issues are not important. They often stop asking or complaining and suffer in silence. Women deserve to have sexuality issues addressed as aggressively as pain or nausea or vomiting. All of these are quality of life issues. Encourage your partner to discuss problems and ask for written information. Contact the organizations listed in the resource section of this book for additional information.

SURGICAL IMPACT ON SEXUALITY

For years, the literature has indicated that the major sexual obstacle after breast cancer is the changed body image from surgery that women experience. However, it seems not to be the major cause for most women. Approximately 50 percent of all breast surgeries are lumpectomy procedures, causing little alteration in physical self-image. Mastectomy patients are having reconstruction at higher rates to restore their body image, unlike women years ago who only had access to a prosthesis to restore their body image. However, with lumpectomy, mastectomy, or reconstruction, the surgical scar and the new body image needs to be shared with the sexual partner.

VIEWING THE SCAR

- When focus group members were asked how long it was before their partners viewed their changed body images, 75% replied that it was within days after surgery.

- When asked how they perceived their partners' response when viewing the scar for the first time, an overwhelming majority, 80%, reported their partners were accepting and supportive.

- 15% reported a neutral response.

- 6% reported that they perceived their response as negative.

- 6% of women in these focus groups reported that their partners had never seen their scar. These women still dress or undress behind closed doors or in the dark.

In Chapter 12 we discussed that one of the potential roadblocks to restoring the sexual relationship may be viewing the surgical scar area.

If a woman accepts her new body image and, more importantly, feels that you do, the sexual relationship suffers only temporary effects and there is no future impact on sexual functioning after the stress and fatigue from surgery are over.

You may notice your sexual relationship changing during the diagnostic and surgical period when the stress is overwhelming for both of you. Sexual feelings are naturally diminished during high periods of stress. However, during periods of stress the need for emotional closeness increases. Most women express that they really need and want more touching, hugging, and emotional closeness during this stressful period. But they often don't know how to express this or are afraid to ask. You may also feel unsure about how to respond and find yourself withdrawing. Do not allow walls of silence and emotional isolation to separate you from your partner and diminish your physical closeness during this time because you are not sure how to treat her. Let her know you still desire to be close and to touch without sexual expectations or demands. Tell her that you would like for her to take the lead in letting you know when she is emotionally and physically ready to resume physical intercourse.

What may change during the post surgical period is how she feels about herself and how she views her attractiveness to you as a sexual partner. You must let her hear and be assured that her reshaped body image has not changed how you see her—that her true beauty, sexuality and attractiveness are just as strong for you now as they were before her surgery. This is essential for the normal resumption of the sexual relationship.

Although it may sound silly, it is important to know that cancer cannot be "caught" from a

SEXUAL FREQUENCY

Focus group responses to sexual frequency after taking chemotherapy showed that:

- 14% reported experiencing no change
- 4% experiencing increased frequency
- 82%, the overwhelming majority— reported **decreased** frequency.

When asked, "did your partner interpret the changes in your sex drive to a personal lack of interest or desire for the relationship?"

- 22% reported that their partners felt they had lost interest in them
- 22% reported they didn't know
- 56% reported that their partners did not interpret the change as such.

This indicates that as a supportive partner you need to make sure she knows that even though there are changes in sexuality, this does not diminish your love or attraction for her.

partner during the sexual relationship. There is no reason that a sexual relationship should not continue in the same manner as before the cancer diagnosis.

When can you resume intercourse after breast cancer surgery? As soon as the two of you feel you would like. If no complications arise, the incision should heal in about four weeks following surgery. However, you may resume your sexual relationship before the area is totally healed. The best time to continue is when both of you feel ready. The surgical scar area will naturally be sore or sensitive, but your partner can lead you in how to prevent pain by altering positions to avoid pressure on the breast. Be open in asking her if she has problems with you touching her surgical breast now or in the future. Some women express that the breast is sensitive and prefer it not be touched or stroked. Others express the opposite feeling; they view their partner's avoidance of touching or stroking their surgical breast as a sign of rejection or non-acceptance of her new image. This creates a problem for partners. The only way you can solve this dilemma in your relationship is to ask her what she desires in the area of touch. You may even find that her desires for touching her breast may change, especially after sensitivity is diminished. The best advice for a good relationship is continued communication about the subject.

RADIATION THERAPY IMPACT ON SEXUALITY

Radiation therapy to the breast area ranges from 5 to 7 weeks of daily treatment (Monday through Friday). If the patient is not getting chemotherapy, radiation starts several weeks after breast surgery or when the incision is healed. If she is having chemotherapy, radiation usually follows the chemotherapy.

During radiation treatments, your partner is not radioactive and sexual contact can continue. However, you may notice that she may experience increased fatigue during treatments, resulting in diminished sexual interest. When radiation treatments are completed, you will find there is no lasting impact on the sexual relationship when her energy returns. The continued fatigue problem is mainly because of chemotherapy.

The side effects of radiation therapy to the breast are redness and tenderness, much like slight sunburn. The breast may swell slightly (edema) during therapy but this usually diminishes over several months to a year after treatment. The patient may feel less sensation in the breast when touched and may notice that the skin of the breast feels slightly increased in thickness. The entire breast may feel firmer, with the skin appearing slightly tanned.

CHEMOTHERAPY IMPACT ON SEXUALITY

If additional treatments with chemotherapy are required, sexuality changes become more of a long-term challenge because of the impact of the drugs. Most chemotherapy teaching is about the well-known side effects of fatigue, nausea, vomiting, and hair loss. Very few couples are forewarned about the impact on their sexual functioning, other than the potential for infertility if the woman is premenopausal. The problem is that chemotherapy most often causes instant menopause in premenopausal women, and increases menopausal side effects for menopausal women.

Menopause caused by chemotherapy is different because it occurs suddenly, unlike normal menopause that occurs over years. The symptoms with chemically induced menopause are more intense because the drugs diminish the hormones made in the ovaries and the adrenal glands. Normal menopause causes a reduction in the ovarian hormones of estrogens, progesterone, and eventually testosterone; but the adrenal glands continue to supply some hormones, causing symptoms to be less severe.

The other important factor to understand is the production of testosterone. Testosterone is predominately a male hormone, but females also make testosterone in the ovaries and convert hormones made by the adrenal gland. Testosterone is the hormone that produces sexual desire and the ability to experience an orgasm, as well as governs the intensity of the orgasm. When a woman takes chemotherapy, she has an instant reduction of all female hormones along with testosterone from both the ovaries and adrenal glands. Side effects of the reduction of estrogen and progesterone are very apparent—hot flashes, night sweats, mood changes, and vaginal dryness. However, the side effects of testosterone reduction are seldom recognized and are often ignored. Because the symptoms are experienced by the patient and impact only her and her partner, they are very rarely addressed. By understanding all of these changes, their causes, and interventions to reduce side effects, your relationship with your partner should not suffer but thrive because of your supportive attitude.

FATIGUE

Obviously, her energy level will be low, and she will not feel like doing much of anything for several days or weeks after each treatment because of lowered blood counts causing fatigue. Fatigue will vary with the type of drugs she receives. Ask her physician about the drugs and expected levels of fatigue. Fatigue has a cumulative effect, increasing as treatment progresses. Encourage her to get additional rest by taking naps or sleeping in when possible. Reduce as many of the tasks of daily living as possible during highest levels of fatigue. Take the initiative to divide household responsibilities among family members or even consider hiring help during this time. Most women are least fatigued the week before treatment. This is the time to plan activities requiring more energy. She may be physically and emotionally exhausted during treatment, but this is all temporary. Be sure that her meals are nutritionally adequate; good nutrition is required to build new cells to replace those that chemotherapy destroys. She may be too tired to prepare nutritionally balanced meals and may need help in this area. Treatments will end, blood counts will increase, and energy will return gradually. It is important to know that the return of energy does not happen in days or weeks when treatment is completed, but requires months, and some women even say a year passed before their normal levels of energy returned.

NAUSEA AND VOMITING

Nausea and vomiting used to be major side effects of chemotherapy, but with new drugs in most cases it can be controlled. It is

> ### FATIGUE
>
> Women participating in the sexuality study indicated their energy level at the time of diagnosis at 7.6 (1 = no energy, 10 = high energy).
>
> When asked how chemotherapy impacted their energy levels:
>
> - 62% reported a decrease from their baseline energy during treatments
>
> - 40% reported a decrease six months after completion of treatments
>
> - 22% reported a continued reduction one-year post treatments.
>
> So, continue to be supportive, protecting her energy expenditure on non-essential activities, knowing that recovery is a gradual process, not an instantaneous occurrence after the last treatment.

important that nausea and vomiting be controlled because this increases fatigue, causes nutrition to be decreased, and increases the potential for electrolyte imbalances. Report any uncontrolled nausea or vomiting to your healthcare team.

MOOD SWINGS

When women lose their estrogen, through natural or chemical menopause, one of the first things they notice is a change in their emotions. Before menopause, this is experienced the few days before their menstrual period and referred to as premenstrual syndrome (PMS). Families are well aware that this time is emotionally different in women. PMS occurs when estrogen and progesterone fall to their lowest levels to allow menstruation. During these few days, increased moodiness, tearfulness, nervousness, and outbursts of anger are common symptoms in many women. The same symptoms occur during reduction of female hormones from chemotherapy. A sad fact is that women are often made to feel that their unstable emotions are caused because they are not "handling cancer" well or that they are depressed.

The fact is, their bodies are thrown into the same emotional limbo as PMS, but it remains day after day because the hormones do not return to reverse the withdrawal. This emotional roller coaster is caused by the chemotherapy drugs and not the patient's emotional weakness or ability to "handle cancer."

It is almost a certainty that mood changes will occur during treatments. The reduction of the female hormones caused by treatment may cause wide fluctuations in her moods. She may swing from normal to sad, then to angry, then to depressed, all with no apparent cause. It is important to understand that she, like you, dislikes the changes she experiences. Relating to her mood swings in an understanding manner, realizing the cause, and not interpreting this as a sign of a diminishing relationship is important.

When the cause of their emotional change is explained to patients, they often break into tears, just from having someone recognize and explain the reason for the mental changes they have endured. As a support partner, recognizing that this is one of the most difficult challenges for women is a great gift of support. The emotional battle they face is not a choice, but a side effect of treatments.

What can a woman do about her mood swings? She can discuss the problems with her physician and ask for a medication called an SSRI (Selected Serotonin Reuptake Inhibitor), which increases the levels of serotonin that elevate mood. The brand names are Celexa, Paxil, Prozac, Zoloft, Lexapro and Luvox. The great thing about these drugs is that they have also proven successful in reducing hot flashes and nervousness and decreasing insomnia.

MOOD SWINGS

Participants in focus groups reported an increase in emotional mood swings:

- 55% increase in mood swings during treatment

- 42% increase six months after treatment ended

- 19% increase at one year after completing treatment

Mood changes after chemotherapy are an expected side effect and vary in degrees of intensity.

VAGINAL DRYNESS
AND PAINFUL INTERCOURSE

Hormonal changes cause the vagina to have less lubrication, resulting in vaginal dryness. Estrogen is the hormone that causes the wall of the vagina to be soft and pliable. With the reduction in estrogen, the vagina becomes very dry. Along with the dryness, the vagina will not lubricate adequately during sexual arousal. If this problem is not understood or corrected, these problems can result in painful intercourse, and possibly a small amount of bleeding after intercourse. Painful intercourse is not pleasant and bleeding can scare both partners. There are interventions that can help with dryness and painful intercourse. There are two types of over-the-counter interventions. One is a vaginal mois-ture-replenishing product in the pharmacy (Replens® or Vagisil®) designed to maintain the moisture in the vagina. Vaginal moisturiz-ers are applied inside the vagina on a regular basis, several times a week, to restore and hold moisture. They are like a moisturizer applied to the face to keep moisture in. They are not designed as a lubricant before intercourse.

The other over-the-counter intervention is a vaginal lubricant. This is applied prior to inter-course to increase lubrication. Astroglide® is highly recommended by patients as being the most like natural lubrication. Vaseline® can promote vaginal infections and should not be used as a lubricant for intercourse. The female should generously apply the lubricant in the vagina and on the outside on the vaginal lips. It can also be applied to the partner to increase lubrication. It is important that the lubricant be reapplied as needed during intercourse.

It is very important for a support partner to know that this vaginal dryness is not from lack of desire from the patient, but from the inability of the walls of the vagina to lubricate caused by the chemical menopause. Often, partners take this reduction of vaginal lubrication as a lack of desire for them as a sexual partner and feel rejected. Some partners feel that the use of lubricant is a sign that they are not sexually stimulating to their partner. Neither is true. Lack of vaginal

---

VAGINAL DRYNESS

Vaginal dryness from chemotherapy was reported to increase:

- 123% during treatment

- 134% six months after treatment ended

- 160% one year after completion of treatments

PAINFUL INTERCOURSE

Painful intercourse from vaginal dryness increased:

- 126% during treatment

- 137% six months after treatment

- 149% one year after treatment completion

These figures reveal that vaginal dryness with the potential to cause painful intercourse increases after treatment is completed. Therefore, couples should be prepared to deal with the lingering side effects.

lubrication is caused by chemical menopause. This is something the patient cannot control. When support partners express their support and encourage use of a lubricant for intercourse, this greatly reduces the anxiety of the patient.

Vaginal dryness is not only uncomfortable; it can also cause itching from dryness. The dryness of the vaginal tissues can also set up an environment for irritating or painful vaginal infections that interfere with sexual pleasure. Any itching or swelling should be reported to the healthcare team for a vaginal infection evaluation. Infections may be caused by an overgrowth of bacteria that causes a thin, gray discharge that has a fishy odor. A fungus (Candida albicans) normally found in the body can experience an overgrowth (often caused by antibiotics) causing a discharge that has a thick, white (cottage cheese like) clumps that cause itching accompanied with internal and external swelling. Both of these vaginal infections can easily be treated with medications.

WHAT CAN WOMEN DO ABOUT VAGINAL DRYNESS
During natural menopause, women are offered oral or transdermal (patch applied to skin) hormone replacement therapy to relieve their symptoms. During breast cancer treatment, at this time, this is usually not an option. However, after treatment is completed, if the vaginal dryness continues even though vaginal moisturizers and lubricants are used, discuss other options with your healthcare provider. The first option would be estrogen vaginal cream applied inside the vagina and on the external vaginal lips or Vagifem®, an estrogen tablet that is inserted into the vagina. Another option is a vaginal ring of estradiol (Estring®) that is inserted into the vagina and remains in place for three months, slowly releasing the drug before replacement is needed. These localized estrogens relieve vaginal dryness, and decrease urinary symptoms. After several months the vagina increases in moisture and elasticity, making intercourse far more comfortable.

URINARY PROBLEMS
When estrogen levels are reduced a common side effect is urinary symptoms. Estrogen receptors are found in the lining of the urinary bladder and tubes. When estrogen levels are low the lining becomes thinner and some women experience burning during urination, urinary urgency, and urinary stress incontinence (loss of urine when walking fast, running, or sneezing). They find holding their urine difficult and often a source of embarrassment. The use of estrogen vaginal cream or Estring will also greatly reduce these symptoms.

ORGASM ABILITY

After treatment with chemotherapy the ability to experience an orgasm during intercourse is reduced for most women. However, a small percentage of women will not suffer this side effect. Hormonal reduction usually continues to create problems for those women who remain in a permanent menopausal state. It can cause an inability to experience an orgasm or reduce the intensity of orgasm if one is experienced. Sexual arousal is also a challenge. One woman in the focus group described her sexual desire after chemotherapy as "that of an 11 year old girl." Diminished sexual interest—sexual thoughts, sexual arousal, and orgasm—are all common side effects of chemotherapy.

It is important to understand that the loss of testosterone—the hormone that causes interest, arousal and orgasm—is the basic problem. What can be done about these side effects? The testosterone can be brought back into normal range by a trained, experienced healthcare provider who understands the complexity of hormonal balance. Many healthcare providers are completely unaware of this intervention. Some contend that they don't know if it is safe. However, those women who have had their levels brought back into therapeutic range with local creams applied to the vaginal area, report that this brought back the sexual quality of life they enjoyed before treatment. Your partner can ask her healthcare team if they check hormonal levels or supplement testosterone. If not, contact the International Academy of Compounding Pharmacists (800-927-4227) and ask for the nearest compounding pharmacy. Your local pharmacy can refer you to the providers in your area who are skilled at testing levels of existing testosterone, and prescribing testosterone cream to be applied to the vaginal area to bring levels back to normal.

SEXUAL INTEREST

Prior to diagnosis:

- 88% of women reported having sexual thoughts and fantasies

- 32% had sexual thoughts and fantasies during treatments

- 41% reported sexual thoughts and fantasies one year after treatment completion

When questioned about the need for extra time to achieve sexual arousal:

- 86% replied that the time required had increased

- 49% reported decreased nipple sensitivity from sexual arousal

- 80% reported lack of vaginal lubrication

One patient, after years of frustration with her lack of libido, called the national number and found a local healthcare provider. She received her prescription for the testosterone cream and after two weeks e-mailed me to say that she had not had any results. My advice was to be patient and continue the use. I received an email after five weeks saying, "My libido is back! This is the best-kept secret in the entire world. Every patient needs to know that there is hope." Return of libido after replacement therapy is used ranges from 2 - 12 weeks.

Return of libido is a quality of life issue. It has nothing to do with life and death issues and for this reason may be ignored. For some couples, return of libido is important to their quality of life. Yet, for others, this is not an issue of importance. Only the two of you can decide what is best for your relationship. There are no right or wrong answers, only what best meets your needs as a couple. It you find that this is an important issue, keep seeking a healthcare provider that addresses your problems, offers interventions, and works to improve your quality of life.

ORGASM ABILITY					
Orgasm	Never	Rarely	Occasionally	Most of Time	All the Time
Before Treatment	1%	8%	19%	55%	17%
During Treatment	24%	27%	28%	16%	5%
One Year After Treatment	10%	23%	29%	30%	9%

Before treatment, 72 percent of women would experience orgasms, varying from most to all of the time. During treatment this fell to 21 percent. Following completion of treatment, this number rose only slightly to 39 percent, translating into a 54 percent reduction in ability to experience orgasms most or all of the time, one year after treatment.

The Orgasm Gap

Males and females have a natural difference in the time between sexual arousal and when orgasm occurs. Dr. Phil McGraw, Ph.D. in his book *Relationship Rescue* states:

"The male's sexual cycle starting at the contemplation of sex through erection, orgasm and loss of erection lasts an average of 2.8 minutes. (see following illustration) Contrasting this to the female's response curve, which builds more gradually and then plateaus at around seven minutes. Her entire cycle lasts approximately thirteen minutes. The problem is that clitoral dilation and vaginal lubrication usually do not occur until several minutes after the males' cycle is completed. Clearly, you can do the math as well as I can. If the males' cycle lasts 2.8 minutes and the females cycle lasts 13 minutes, then we have a ten-minute gap in compatibility."

Average Male & Female Orgasm Cycles

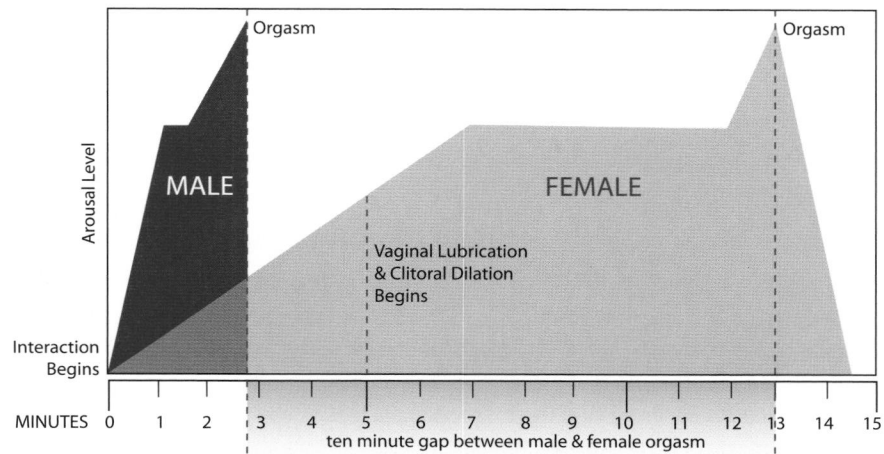

You can see from this data, extensive foreplay is needed if a female partner is to experience orgasm. Wellbutrin, an anti-depressant, has proven helpful in increasing libido and the ability to have an orgasm for some women.

Fatigue from surgery, radiation and chemotherapy treatments can alter sexual arousal even more. Wise planning is needed for mutual satisfaction.

Dr. Charles Carver, a professor of psychology at the University of Miami, conducted a study of 240 breast cancer surgical patients involved in long-term relationships and its impact on their relationship with their partner. When asked about their first sexual encounter after surgery the study concluded, "The higher women rated the quality of their first sexual experience after surgery, the greater their feelings of femininity and attractiveness, the less emotional distress they experienced and the more satisfied with their future relationship." Women also reported that their perception of their sexual desirability to their partner came primarily from their partner expressing and initiating sex and the frequency of the sexual contact.

> *We were both emotionally drained. I had to give my mate a chance to regroup. The actual sexual act could wait. However, we both needed touching, cuddling and holding each other.*
> *It was important that I tell her I still found her attractive. I allowed her to set the guidelines on how and when the sexual relationship would be resumed.*
>
> **—AL BARRINEAU**
> **SUPPORT PARTNER**

TIPS FOR RESUMING THE SEXUAL RELATIONSHIP:

Communicating your continued attraction to her as a sexual partner is the most important foundation for resuming a successful sexual relationship. Find as many ways as possible to convey this message. Say it. Write notes. Send cards. Touch her. Go on special dates together, no matter how simple they may be.

- View the incision area soon after surgery and get this major obstacle to sexual functioning out of the way.

- Verbalize your desire for the resumption of the relationship when she feels ready.

- If surgery is the only treatment, sexually normalcy is solely based on how she views her body image and how she thinks you view her as a sexual partner. Surgery will not impact and cause reduction in the female hormones causing the multitude of symptoms discussed. The sexual relationship can be resumed as soon as is mutually desired. Remember to communicate about the potential tenderness of the surgical breast and what is most comfortable to your partner.

- If radiation therapy follows surgery and chemotherapy treatments are not required, an added obstacle may be the fatigue experienced by some women. This fatigue is not debilitating, but simply a tired feeling that can be helped by additional rest. Some women find going for treatments daily for weeks is emotionally stressful, and this emotional stress can impact hormonal levels that can reduce desire. The best advice is to openly communicate your desire to resume sexual intercourse when she feels ready, but continue to be physically and emotionally close by continuing to touch and hold her.

- For women who have chemotherapy, the challenge is far greater, as we have discussed. You will face additional challenges with addressing hair loss (alopecia), which has proven more difficult for women than dealing with the surgical changes of the breast. Fatigue from chemotherapy may be physically overwhelming during treatments for some women, while others may simply feel tired. Chemotherapy women suffer a double blow to their self-image (surgery and chemotherapy) and need extra assurance that they remain sexually attractive as a partner.

- Plan a time when her energy is at its highest to resume a sexual relationship. The week or several days before her next chemo treatment is a good choice.

- Plan a special time for closeness—a special date, dinner, movie, or whatever she enjoys.

- Allow adequate time to touch and stroke her body. Sexual arousal will be slower and foreplay may need to be longer because of the reduction of female hormones.

- Don't force or ask her to remove her gown or prosthesis if she does not feel comfortable. This may cause her to withdraw emotionally. Some women said that it took several months before they really felt free to participate in intercourse without their scar area covered. Others admitted never wanting to have sexual intercourse without their scar area covered, even though the partner had seen the incision. Removing their clothing resulted in reducing her sexual feelings. Do what she feels is comfortable.

- Prepare for sexual relations by having adequate amounts of a water-based lubricant available. Some women find that when their partners apply the lubricant, it is sexually arousing. Simply ask what she prefers.

- During treatment with chemotherapy, it is recommended that you use latex condoms.

- After intercourse, remain close and continue to touch her in a loving way. Assure her that she is still the same loving partner and gives you the same pleasure.

As in all other areas of the breast cancer experience, women and their partners will react differently to each situation. Use these tips as suggestions only. Some partners have said that their sexual relationships were even more gratifying after the cancer experience. Recognizing and understanding that the changes following surgery and treatments are a normal part of the recovery process will make you a more sensitive partner. If problems do arise at a later date and you have difficulty working through the changes, trained sexuality counselors are available in most cancer treatment centers or in your community.

REMEMBER

SURGERY AND RADIATION THERAPY CAUSE ONLY TEMPORARY CHANGES IN SEXUAL FUNCTIONING

CHEMOTHERAPY CAN CAUSE VARYING LEVELS OF EFFECTS IMPACTING SEXUALITY, FOR WHICH YOU NEED TO UNDERSTAND AND PREPARE TO SUPPORT YOUR PARTNER IN FINDING APPROPRIATE INTERVENTIONS.

RESUMPTION OF THE SEXUAL RELATIONSHIP NEEDS TO BE APPROACHED WITH SENSITIVITY AND PLANNING.

YOUR UNDERSTANDING OF THE CHANGES SHE FACES IS NECESSARY FOR THE SEXUAL RELATIONSHIP TO REMAIN HEALTHY.

SUPPORT PARTNERS

SUPPORT PARTNERS
HAVE A DUAL ROLE.

OUTWARDLY YOU MUST BE
EMPATHIC, CARING,
AVAILABLE AND SUPPORTIVE
OF THE ONE YOU LOVE.

INSIDE, YOUR HEART
MAY BE BREAKING;
YOU MAY STRUGGLE
WITH FEARS AND OFTEN FEEL
OVERWHELMED WITH DESPAIR.

SUPPORT PARTNERS HURT TOO.
YOU ALSO NEED TO FIND
A SAFE PLACE WHERE THE ROLES
ARE REVERSED AND
YOU RECEIVE THE SUPPORT
YOU NEED.

— JUDY KNEECE

FUTURE FERTILITY

One of the issues least thought about during a cancer diagnosis is the impact of cancer treatments from chemotherapy and hormonal therapy on future fertility. Most thoughts naturally focus on the patient and getting the most appropriate treatment for her cancer. However, one of the most important issues for younger couples who have not had or completed having their family is the potential impact on their future fertility. It is essential for couples to ask these questions to protect or plan future alternative methods. This chapter will briefly discuss these important issues regarding future fertility.

For women, infertility is the inability to start or maintain a pregnancy. Infertility can occur because of the inability of the ovaries to produce mature eggs (oocytes) for ovulation, or from the inability of the body to successfully allow implantation of a fertilized egg into the uterine wall or maintain its growth after implantation.

WOMEN AND THE FERTILITY CYCLE

When a woman is born, she has all of the eggs she will ever have and does not produce more. When the female hormones gear up at puberty she experiences the development of secondary sex characteristics such as pubic hair, breasts, and menstruation. Eventually, the menstrual cycles are accompanied by the release of a

> *We were newlyweds when Anna was diagnosed; however, that did not mean that the diagnosis did not bring fears about our future as parents. We shared the intense fear that chemotherapy had the potential to rob us of the anticipated joy of having children one day. We still wrestle with the fear that 'if we could have children today, what would happen if Anna had a recurrence?'*
>
> **—BRIAN CLUXTON**
> **SUPPORT PARTNER**

mature egg at mid-cycle (ovulation) ready for fertilization by the male sperm. If conception does not occur, or if the fertilized egg does not successfully implant into the uterine wall, the prepared ovarian wall sloughs off, evidenced by the menstrual flow. The entire process begins again for another monthly cycle. Each full cycle averages from 28 – 32 days. Each ovulation reduces the amount of stored eggs. Eventually the supply of eggs that mature is reduced, ovulation ceases, hormones decrease to pre-menstrual levels, and eventually the menstrual periods stop. This cessation of ovarian function along with the loss of fertility is called menopause. With menopause comes symptoms, not only of infertility, but most often including hot flashes, vaginal dryness, changes in moods, urinary changes, and other menopausal symptoms.

CHEMOTHERAPY: POTENTIAL IMPACT ON FERTILITY

Surgery has no effect on fertility, other than creating stress which causes temporary changes in the hormonal balance that may temporarily alter ovulation and possibly menstruation. This usually resolves itself in several months. Radiation therapy to the breast by itself has only temporary effects, similar to surgery—stress and fatigue may alter hormonal functioning temporally, if at all. The major cause of infertility comes from chemotherapy.

Chemotherapy drugs used to treat cancer work by killing rapidly dividing cells throughout the body. Chemotherapy drugs are cytotoxic (cyto=cell, toxic=poison). These drugs kill cancer cells, but in the process also kill healthy, rapidly dividing cells as well. Shortly after chemotherapy administration, women notice hormonal changes in their body. A large majority of women suffer irregular or complete cessation of periods during treatment. Factors that determine the extent of their side effects and may also impact their future infertility are based on the patient's age, drug type, or drug combinations that may compound the effect of toxicity on the body. It is very difficult for an oncologist to accurately predict who will suffer side effects involving their hormonal functioning. Fertility may return after the drugs are discontinued for some women, but for others their infertility may be permanent.

There are facts that are known to help in fertility prediction:

The nearer a patient is to menopause, the less likely she is to have hormonal function (menstruation and ovulation) return. The younger a woman, the more likely hormonal function will return.

A class of drugs, called alkylating agents, have a more destructive affect on hormonal function. The most common one used in breast cancer treatment is cyclophosphamide (Cytoxan). Other drugs that increase infertility in this category are melphalan (Alkeran) and busulfan (Myleran). Cisplatin (Platinol) is usually considered an alkylating agent even though it works differently than the others in this category and also impacts fertility.

ADDRESSING ISSUES OF FERTILITY

Since physicians cannot predict with absolute certainty whose fertility can be permanently affected, there are steps to take to preserve your mate's future ability to have children.

- The most essential step is telling your healthcare team before treatments that having children is top priority when making treatment decisions.
- Ask your healthcare team to discuss treatment recommendations and their potential for causing infertility.
- Ask for written information on the subject of chemotherapy and fertility.
- Ask for a referral to a specialist in the area of fertility if you still have questions or concerns.
- Ask for treatment protocols to be used that reduce potential for infertility.
- Explore alternative fertility preservation options.

ALTERNATIVE FERTILITY PRESERVATION OPTIONS:

Embryo Freezing

Hormones (like Tamoxifen, safe in breast cancer) are used to stimulate egg production. Mature eggs are removed by a physician in a minor surgical procedure, fertilized in vitro (in a glass test tube) with sperm, frozen for future use, and then stored. This procedure is called in-vitro fertilization (IVF). Pregnancy rates average 10 – 25 percent with each frozen embryo.

Egg (Oocyte) Freezing

Hormones (like Tamoxifen) are used to stimulate egg production. Mature eggs are retrieved by the physician, frozen for future use, and then stored without being fertilized. This method is new and at present has an estimated pregnancy success rate of 3 percent.

Research in Progress: Ovarian Retrieval and Transplantation

Ovaries are surgically removed by laparoscopy (small incision through abdomen), divided into small strips, frozen, and later transplanted back into the body when fertility is desired. Drugs are given to stimulate ovulation. Some researchers call the process ovarian grafting. This method is experimental but appears to have potential for women who have chemotherapy that will damage their ovaries. Check with your healthcare team on the progress of this research.

The procedures for fertility preservation are expensive and usually require several months for egg retrieval, which may delay treatments. At this time, most of the cost is not covered by insurance. During breast cancer decisions, this adds another difficult choice for some couples that still desire to have a family of their own. But this is an important consideration if future fertility is desired. It is also important to know that some cancers require immediate attention. One is inflammatory carcinoma, a cancer that is already advanced because of involvement of the lymphatic system and which requires that treatment start within days of diagnosis. Discuss with your physician whether any type of delay would reduce her chances for survival.

Optional Parenthood Choices:

Some couples find that their main priority during the diagnostic period is the patient receiving optimal treatment for her cancer. Fertility is not the prominent issue at this time. There are other methods that are still optional:

- Using donor eggs, if fertility does not return
- Using a surrogate mother
- Adoption

FACTS ABOUT PREGNANCY AFTER BREAST CANCER:

- Pregnancy does not seem to reduce patient survival or trigger recurrence
- Women who have had systemic chemotherapy have been able to conceive and deliver healthy, normal children with the chance of birth defects near that of the normal untreated population
- Some physicians suggest that a couple wait six months before pregnancy is attempted after regular menstrual periods return. Ask your physician about their guidelines

QUESTIONS FOR HEALTHCARE TEAM IF CHEMOTHERAPY IS TREATMENT OPTION:

- What is the predicted impact on fertility from the drugs?
- What percentage of women who take these drugs experience permanent infertility?
- Are there drugs with less potential for infertility that can be used?
- What options do we have to preserve our fertility?
- Do you make referrals to physicians specializing in fertility preservation, if we desire one?
- If we decide to pursue embryo freezing as an option, will the time required to collect the eggs impact her survival outcomes by delaying treatment for several months or so?
- If her fertility returns, how long do you suggest we wait before she attempts pregnancy?

REMEMBER

FUTURE FERTILITY IS AN ISSUE THAT MIGHT NOT BE DISCUSSED BY YOUR HEALTHCARE TEAM IF YOU DO NOT BRING UP THE SUBJECT.

IF FUTURE FERTILITY IS IMPORTANT, ASK FOR INFORMATION AND A REFERRAL TO A FERTILITY SPECIALIST TO DISCUSS OPTIONS BEST SUITED FOR YOUR PARTNER.

SUPPORT PARTNERS

ARE SHELTERS OF SAFETY FOR

THE ONE THEY LOVE

WHEN IN CRISIS.

THEY ARE A SAFE PLACE

TO FALL, WHEN THE WORLD

COMES TUMBLING IN.

IN THEIR PRESENCE THEY FEEL

THE SAFETY OF TRUST,

UNDERSTANDING AND FIND

UNCONDITIONAL LOVE.

— JUDY KNEECE

HER EMOTIONAL ADJUSTMENT TO BREAST CANCER

B reast cancer can serve as a "wake-up call" to life. In one woman's words, "I realized that I was not going to live forever when I received my diagnosis. I had never stopped to think about it before! But now I live every day to the fullest. No longer will I be a slave to those things in life that were of no consequence." A new lease on life, a desire to make every day and minute count, is often the result of the cancer experience.

A year after her surgery one patient reminisced, "Breast cancer was the worst thing that ever happened to me and the best thing that ever happened to me. Even though I hated every change my cancer caused my family to go through, as I reflect, it has brought us a greater degree of happiness and love, and today I would not trade the experience." Many patients and families report a greater degree of happiness after breast cancer because they decided to concentrate on happiness rather than things. Facing the dreaded enemy caused them to refocus their priorities.

> *Breast cancer threatened our relationship. We are taking advantage of our second chance. We've fallen in love all over again. I've seen my wife blossom before my eyes.*
>
> **—AL BARRINEAU**
> **SUPPORT PARTNER**

This is an excellent time to encourage your mate to do some things she has always wanted to do but did not take the time for. Encourage her to use breast cancer as the reason to do the things she dreams of and not as an excuse not to. Support her in beginning a hobby, taking a class, getting a pet, planting a flower garden, changing careers, going back to school, becoming a volunteer or planning a trip—whatever she has an interest in doing. A sense of accomplishment will provide a helpful environment for emotional and physical recovery.

WHEN EMOTIONAL ADJUSTMENT BECOMES DIFFICULT

By the time most women complete their treatments they have adjusted emotionally to the experience and are putting their lives back into a normal routine. Occasionally, someone has difficulty returning to normal. Even though things are physically going well, and life is ready to return to a normal routine, emotionally, they don't want to move forward and rejoin the family. They seem to be locked into distrust and fear of the future. They don't look forward to the days, months, or years ahead. They have lost interest in the things that they once found joyful. Their laughter has been silenced. They find it difficult to plan. They withdraw from family and friends, avoiding social activities when possible. They prefer to spend their time sleeping or in solitude. Some overeat and some have lost their pleasure in food. Some resort to the overuse of alcohol or drugs to numb their pain. Occasionally, they may even express that life is not worth living any longer. Somehow, the person you knew before her diagnosis has not come back to you emotionally. She has changed greatly.

If you recognize these symptoms in the one you love, you will need to alert someone on the healthcare team. Being the person closest to the patient, you will be able to accurately recognize if your mate is continuing to have problems coping. If this should occur, inform your primary care physician and ask for a referral to a professional counselor. Depressed people may not even recognize that they are depressed.

Even if they do, some patients do not consider their mood disturbances a concern that they should take to the physician. They sometimes think that continuing sad feelings after **cancer are normal, but they are not**. As a support partner, your close relationship to the patient allows an understanding of what is normal behavior for the patient and what is not. The first step is to understand how to distinguish a **normal reactive depression** from a **clinical depression.**

> *My wife had a history of clinical depression so we had an added area of concern as to how she would handle all of this. She did great in the beginning, but, after chemotherapy, a new kind of tears and withdrawal started. We then tried one-to-one counseling and a breast cancer support group. Encouraging, talking with, crying with and receiving encouragement from others walking in the same shoes helped her tremendously.*
>
> **—AL BARRINEAU**
> **SUPPORT PARTNER**

DISTINGUISHING NORMAL DEPRESSION FROM CLINICAL DEPRESSION

Normal depression after a loss is an expected reaction. It is described as "feeling blue" or "feeling down" when one has lost something that is valuable to them physically or emotionally. Breast cancer is certainly a loss to a woman. It is normal for her to cry and feel down at the time of diagnosis and at the beginning of or during treatment. However, during this time, the person may feel sad but can still enjoy and look forward to parts of her life, such as a family gathering, a movie, or seeing a child, grandchild or friend. She still reaches out and shares life's joys and sorrows with those around her.

Clinical depression is severe depression that causes many physical and emotional changes and needs the intervention of a professional. Clinical depression is often manifested by:

- Continuous feeling of sadness (after diagnosis, treatments)
- Social withdrawal from family and friends
- Feelings of worthlessness
- Excessive feelings of guilt
- Excessive feelings of fearfulness
- Feelings of hopelessness about the future
- Being very slow in physical movement or speech
- Feeling constantly jittery or nervous
- Low energy level; may feel tired all the time
- Inability to make decisions
- Negative thinking
- Imaginary health problems
- Lack of interest in food or eating excessively
- Disinterest in work or day-to-day activities
- Uninterested in intimacy or sex
- Insomnia (inability to sleep—wakes early or cannot go to sleep) or sleeps too much
- Suicidal thoughts*

*Immediately notify a healthcare professional of suicidal expressions or threats.

> *Breast cancer was a life-changing event for us. We decided not to brush it under the rug; but instead look for how we could it turn it into a positive experience. Today, we both see life completely different than before her diagnosis; we live more in the present. We decided to use our experience working with other young couples diagnosed with cancer through the Young Survival Coalition.*
>
> **—BRIAN CLUXTON**
> **SUPPORT PARTNER**

If your partner exhibits several (some say five or more) of these symptoms for a period of several weeks or longer, your physician should be notified.

TREATMENT OF DEPRESSION

Depression may be treated in several ways. In some cases, counseling may be all that is needed. Counseling identifies weakness in coping skills and works to strengthen them. Often, talking to an understanding person accomplishes much for a depressed person. However, medication may be needed to assist the process. Anti-depressants are often prescribed and will take approximately two weeks to become effective. Diet and exercise have also been proven to be beneficial to reduce depression and stress. Ask your physician for recommendations. A class of drugs called SSRIs (Selected Serotonin Reuptake Inhibitors) is very effective for relieving depression. The brand names are Celexa, Paxil, Prozac, Zoloft, Lexapro and Luvox. These drugs not only elevate moods, they have also proven successful in reducing hot flashes, nervousness and decreasing insomnia.

It is important that your mate understands that **depression is not a sign of weakness.** It is a legitimate condition that is experienced by many people after a major crisis or loss. Most depression is periodic, and short-term counseling and medication will help through this period of adjustment. Identifying and seeking help is the first step to resolving the problem of depression. If you feel that this may be occurring in your partner, **encourage her to call her physician. If the depression is severe, you may have to notify her physician.** She may lack the emotional energy to reach out for help.

EVENTS WHICH TRIGGER NORMAL REACTIVE DEPRESSION

Post-Treatment Depression

After a major loss, there are periods of normal depression that may be predicted. There is a period of depression that often occurs several weeks after or at the end of treatment when the patient is no longer going to the cancer treatment center on a regular, monthly basis.

One patient recalled, "Somehow I felt while I was getting chemotherapy that they were doing something about my cancer; then all of a sudden I completed my treatments. I thought that this was the time that I had waited for so intensely over the past six months, but to my surprise, I felt frightened. No one was doing anything. I was not seeing anyone. Then the fears overwhelmed me. I didn't know if I could make it on my own. I found myself experiencing many of the sad feelings I had felt at diagnosis, the tears started back. . . . I withdrew emotionally, my appetite left, and I was unable to sleep. But, thankfully, a family member brought my condition to the attention of my physician. I was relieved to know that these feelings happened to many patients at the conclusion of their treatments, and, after talking openly with them, I began to understand."

The conclusion of chemotherapy or radiation therapy treatments is a common time for patients to experience depression. The months of constant contact with the healthcare staff provide a sense of security and socialization for the patient. When treatment ceases and her medical support team is not seen monthly, she becomes very concerned and may feel somewhat alone. Periods of sadness exhibited by the patient are normal and sometimes last for several consecutive days. But, if this time turns into weeks, it is advisable to seek assistance for your loved one.

Knowing this, it is helpful for you as a support partner to plan to spend extra time or plan a special event at the conclusion of her treatments.

Anniversary Depression

Another common time for depression is around the anniversary date of her diagnosis, surgery, or other some events involving the cancer diagnosis. These dates may serve as triggers for an "anniversary reaction" and result in a short period of depression. The date brings back all the memories of the event so clearly that the patient finds herself reliving the event to the point that many of the old feelings return. The result may be a brief period of depression.

One psychiatrist, who had bilateral mastectomies, plans a special event for herself on the day of her original diagnosis for breast cancer. She plans a light workday or, if possible, takes the day off and treats herself. She plans for family members or friends to spend this time with her. Wise planning can help during these expected times of emotional conflict. Yearly regression into many of the old, experienced feelings may happen for years after the event. This is a normal reaction to a traumatic event. Careful planning around these dates to avoid further stress, in addition to your understanding, will help during these times.

Physical Checkup Depression

Return visits to the physician for checkups can also renew many of the anxious, depressive feelings associated with breast cancer. Many women experience high levels of anxiety for several days surrounding their return visits to the physician for checkups. Know that this reaction is normal and allow her these brief periods of emotional regression. Check to see if she needs you to be with her for these checkups. If so, plan to accompany her or arrange to have a friend or family member go with her to the physician. Her greatest fear is that of recurrence and it is most helpful if you both understand and talk about this.

When Treatments End

The breast cancer experience will have changed many things for you and for your mate. Understanding and recognizing some of the major emotional traps of post-treatment depression, anniversary reactions, and return physician visits will allow the two of you to plan wisely to maneuver through the brief emotional storms.

REMEMBER

By the time surgery, treatments, and reconstruction (if chosen) are completed, you both will have been under extended stress. Do not be surprised to find yourself suffering from exhaustion when it is all over. This is a time to plan something special for the two of you to enjoy together. It is also the time you will need to find out what schedule of tests and visits will monitor her health in the future. Mark your calendar and then try to put breast cancer out of your focus for a while.

MANAGING THE FEAR OF RECURRENCE

At a time when the battle with treatment for breast cancer is over and life can resume some sense of normalcy, the fear of recurrence can seem like a dark, black cloud. This fear can rob couples of a sense of safety and poses a great obstacle for happiness, adding much stress to the relationship. This was the most commonly expressed fear by support partners of the patients I worked with in support groups, and the number one fear of breast cancer survivors.

To gain a sense of control over the fear of recurrence, it will be helpful if you take steps to manage it. The first step is to acknowledge your fear. The second step is to know that your mate has the same fear. She, too, has to deal with this fear that robs joy from the future. It will be very helpful if you can face this obstacle as a team. Talking with each other about the need to rationally approach the problem will be the foundation for your plan.

Surgery, chemotherapy and reconstruction were all behind us. Yet, there was a cloud of fear over our lives–recurrence. Finding the proper balance between necessary follow-up care and obsession with recurrence can prove a challenge, especially the first few years. The new appreciation for each other and life itself will be lost if you don't control and deal with your fears.

—AL BARRINEAU
SUPPORT PARTNER

MANAGING THE FEAR OF RECURRENCE

How do you manage the fear of recurrence as a couple? Denial is certainly not the answer. Understand that this is the most common fear of patients and their partners. It is a natural fear.

You are completely normal to feel this fear, as is your partner. In fact, for couples that do not experience this anxiety, there is a danger that they are not dealing with the reality of a breast cancer diagnosis. No one can ever guarantee anyone that there is no more cancer in the future. The greatest problem I have encountered is the fact that most couples do not have an accurate understanding of the realistic risks of recurrence. More often, their fears are exaggerated to a degree far greater than the truth.

There are guidelines, however, that can help predict the risk of recurrence. You need to know these risks. This is the first step to managing fear—finding accurate information. To begin finding truth, you and your mate will need to talk with her physician. You cannot manage what you don't know. This information must come from your mate's healthcare team and not from the media or well-meaning friends. Accurate information is necessary.

MANAGEMENT STRATEGIES FOR FEAR OF RECURRENCE:

Make an appointment with your physician to talk about your mate's particular risks. Some support partners feel a need to talk to the physician in private about their mate's risks. You will need to decide what will best meet your needs. Ask the following questions:

1. What are her risks for recurrence?

Most often, support partners overestimate the risk. You need to know the truth. But, remember to use statistical data as a guideline, not as an absolute fact. Every woman is an individual and does not necessarily fit the statistical tables.

2. How often will she return to you for a checkup?

Return visits for checkups vary. They are usually every three months after treatment and are gradually reduced if no problems arise.

FOCUS GROUP - MAJOR SURVIVOR CHALLENGE

Focus group participants responded to the question of ranking their greatest present challenge from a pre-selected list of potential problems. Participants ranked major challenges as follows:

- Fear of recurrence   56%
- Job loss   4%
- Insurance   7%
- Relationship   8%
- Social/career barriers   2%
- Side effects of treatment   23%

As indicated in the chart above, the fear of recurrence was the overwhelming number one challenge of women in the focus groups. Most couples will find that it is usually one of the main challenges they face after treatment completion.

3. What diagnostic tests do you plan to perform on these checkups?

On return physician visits, a careful history of events since the last visit and a physical exam are performed. Physicians have various schedules on which to perform blood work studies, mammograms, bone scans, liver scans, CT scans, chest x-rays, etc. Ask what scheduled tests are planned as follow-up care. Women are often frightened when they are scheduled for some diagnostic tests. They think the physician is suspicious of a recurrence, when in reality the test is a regularly scheduled follow-up test for all patients.

4. What signs and symptoms do we need to report?

Your physician will tell you the most likely signs of recurrence, according to the type of breast cancer your mate had. Cancers vary in their likelihood of recurring in a specific manner. Your physician can help you know which symptoms need immediate medical attention.

5. What can we do to maximize her recovery?

Ask about diet, exercise, breast self-exam, and medications she should or should not take (example, estrogen-type medications). Physicians will often recommend professionals to work with the patient to learn about diet, exercise programs, and breast self-exam. Encourage your mate to participate in learning, but do not force her. Patients often need a time for emotional retreat and find it stressful to take on any new challenges immediately after treatment is completed.

One of the ways you may help is to offer to participate in some of these recovery strategies. You may both wish to change your dietary habits or start an exercise program together. Breast self-exam is also a good tool to help monitor for recurrence in the remaining breast and the scar area. Some women report that this often causes much stress and they are often fearful to perform their exams. One way you may help is to offer to learn to do the exam for her. One husband reported that his wife was overwhelmed with fear about checking her breasts. "I asked for instructions and I now perform this task for her monthly. ... It is not a bad job! ... In fact, this has been our bonding time in fighting the fear of recurrence together." Look for your own ways to make recovery a partnership.

COMMUNICATING FEARS TO YOUR HEALTHCARE TEAM

Most physicians have a nurse who is qualified to answer many questions by patients and to refer those that need a physician's attention. Identify this person. It is normal to think the first few years that every pain is a sign of recurrence. Managing these fears is best accomplished by communicating with the person who can appropriately evaluate your concerns. Utilize this fear management technique. If you have any questions call and ask this person immediately, rather than worrying and waiting until the next appointment date. Use your healthcare team as your advisor as to whether there is a cause for concern when symptoms arise.

COMMUNICATING WITH YOUR MATE

The next step after getting accurate information from your healthcare team will be the need to build an open, honest relationship with your mate about these concerns. She needs to feel that she can share her physical concerns and fears without "upsetting" you. Women often feel uncomfortable sharing physical symptoms; they don't want to worry anyone. However, you can help monitor her health if she feels free to tell you how she is feeling, or if she has any physical changes occurring.

As we discussed previously, she also needs to have the freedom to verbalize her fears in times in which she is vulnerable—checkups, anniversary dates, and times of depression. Her road to recovery may have some detours through anxiety and days of depression. This is normal. You can help by recognizing these times, allowing her to talk and giving her support.

Help her plan a stress-free schedule, if possible, around anniversary dates and checkups. She will vividly remember these times and your acknowledgment by being supportive will be very helpful to her emotional recovery. Plan a special treat—a meal out, a single flower, a note telling her of your love—to make these times easier. Remember, she is not looking to you for miracles, only for your understanding and support.

> *I consciously choose not to think about recurrence; it is too painful emotionally. Anna monitors her health and follows her doctor's recommendations for followup. We choose to enjoy life today and not dwell on a potential disaster that could be lurking in our future. Personally, I don't think of that as denial, but rather as a healthy way to cope with what you cannot control.*
>
> **—BRIAN CLUXTON**
> **SUPPORT PARTNER**

MANAGING YOUR ANXIETIES

We have been discussing managing fears of recurrence as partners and how you can help your mate by allowing open communication. Yet, a very vital part of your personal fear management is finding someone with whom you can openly share your fears and feelings. These will be found in support groups, friends, professional counselors, and spiritual counselors. Look for these sources of support from those who truly understand and avail yourself of the help they offer. One support partner said, "We need to understand the needs of our mates, but we also need to understand and meet our own needs for support. I found this source in a support group of other mates. That is when I finally managed to get my fears under control. . . . I needed support too."

REMEMBER

"To fight fear, ACT.
To increase fear—wait, put off, postpone."

—DAVID JOSEPH SCHWARTZ

"Fear is conquered by action. When we challenge
our fears, we defeat them. When we grapple with our
difficulties, they lose their hold upon us. When we
dare to face the things which scare us, we open the
door to freedom."

—WYNN ADAMS

"You gain strength, courage, and confidence by every
experience in which you really stop to look fear in the
face. The danger lies in refusing to face the fear, in not
daring to come to grips with it. You must do something
you think you cannot do."

—ELEANOR ROOSEVELT

"Fear can keep us up all night,
but faith makes one fine pillow."

—PHILIP GULLEY

THE FEAR OF
RECURRENCE IS A
JOY ROBBER,
AND YOU AND YOUR MATE
MUST ADDRESS IT WITH
ACCURATE
INFORMATION AND OPEN
COMMUNICATION FOR
OPTIMAL EMOTIONAL
RECOVERY.

ACCURATE INFORMATION
IS OBTAINED BY CONSULTING
WITH THE HEALTHCARE TEAM
CONCERNING RISKS AND
SIGNS AND SYMPTOMS THAT
NEED TO BE REPORTED.

MATES HAVE PREDICTABLE
TIMES WHEN THEIR FEARS OF
RECURRENCE INCREASE—
PHYSICAL CHECKUPS AND
ANNIVERSARY DATES OF
DIAGNOSIS OR
SURGERY/TREATMENT.
WISE PLANNING CAN
REDUCE THE INTENSITY OF
THEIR FEAR.

MATES ARE NOT LOOKING
TO YOU FOR MIRACLES,
ONLY LOVING SUPPORT.

SUPPORTING SOMEONE

WE CANNOT TELL

WHAT MAY HAPPEN TO US

IN THIS STRANGE MEDLEY OF LIFE.

BUT WE CAN DECIDE

WHAT HAPPENS IN US

AND HOW WE TAKE IT,

WHAT WE DO WITH IT,

AND THAT IS WHAT

REALLY COUNTS IN THE END.

HOW TO TAKE THE

RAW STUFF OF LIFE

AND MAKE IT

A THING OF

WORTH AND BEAUTY . . .

THAT IS THE TEST OF LIVING.

— JOSEPH FORT NEWTON

SHARED INSIGHTS ON COPING

W orking as a Breast Health Navigator, I have had the opportunity to observe hundreds of mates as they worked through the breast cancer experience with the ones they loved. It is not an easy task. Being a support partner is one of the most difficult tasks because there is no training and there are very few guidelines to allow you to know if you are doing the right things.

My observations reveal that some partners become so hyper-attentive in their new role that they forget to take care of their own needs as they endeavor to meet all of their mate's physical and emotional needs. Some feel inadequate and fail to try to make things better. They fall into a pattern of denial or avoidance of their mate's crisis and leave the patient to depend on friends or other family members for support. Most often, mates muster all of the emotional muscle available and learn to become the support partner needed by the patient.

In this effort, I have seen wonderful things happen to couples. I have seen relationships grow into a deeper commitment. I have witnessed a new love develop for the partner. One patient shares, "We feel like we did when

> " Finding the proper balance in your life is a challenge, especially in the first few years after diagnosis. The new appreciation for each other and life itself will be lost if you don't control your own fears. Take interest in her emotional as well as physical recovery, but do the same for yourself. You aren't going to be much help to her if you don't take care of yourself. "
>
> —AL BARRINEAU
> SUPPORT PARTNER

we were dating 25 years ago. We can't wait to see each other at the close of the day. Somehow we had gotten so busy we had lost each other in a flurry of careers and activities. Breast cancer gave us back the gift of our love for each other." Many relationships experience this renewal.

Working closely with mates in support groups and as individuals, I had the privilege of listening as they shared the things that made a difference in helping them in this new role as support partner. I asked support partners to share with me their best advice in our effort to make your journey a little easier.

- Acknowledge your mate's and your own emotions. Don't stifle them. Don't try to be too positive; this can be as difficult for your mate as your being depressed.

- Find someone you can trust—someone who understands your needs—and talk with them. We all need support; it makes life easier to bear.

- Gather up-to-date information on the disease and become knowledgeable of the basic decisions that need to be made. Often women are paralyzed with fear and cannot take these steps. Knowledge increases your sense of control and allows you to become partners with the healthcare team.

- Recruit needed help from your family and friends. They want to be helpful and appreciate it when you tell them specifically what your needs are at the time. Don't make them guess.

- Keep organized in your record-keeping. Get a calendar and keep records of appointment dates and treatments received. Ask for copies of bills to file for future reference. This will help when insurance companies and hospitals are billing you for services—often months later.

- Rearrange your previous priorities, realizing it will be for a limited period of time, not forever. A golf game may need to be exchanged for a walk with your mate or an outing to the mall for her emotional support. You may even need to take an occasional "mental health" day from work to take care of your own emotional and physical needs.

- Plan special and fun times for you and your mate together. Often, recreation and fun times are abandoned during treatment, but

> *For us, the whole breast cancer experience has almost been a blessing; I know that is hard for you to believe or even think it's possible right after the diagnosis of the one you love. It takes time, but today we have a closer relationship than ever before. We have learned a lot about our relationship, and I learned a lot about myself that I would not have learned without the experience.*
>
> —BRIAN CLUXTON
> SUPPORT PARTNER

this should not be the case. Be creative in how recreation may have to be changed because of limited amounts of energy, but plan some time of diversion for the two of you. During chemotherapy the best time is the days before her next treatment.

- Seek feedback from your mate. There is a careful balance between communication and silence, withdrawal and over-involvement, separateness and togetherness, attentiveness and emotional distance. Mates have different involvement needs. Be sure that you are not expending too much energy in areas that she may feel are unnecessary.

- Understand normal changes in sexual functioning from surgery, radiation therapy, chemotherapy and hormonal medications and take steps to avoid the obstacles you may have in restoring a sexual relationship. Understanding and communicating is a necessary part for support partners in helping their partners deal with the changes.

- Take care of yourself physically. As your focus changes to your mate's needs during surgery and treatment, be sure that you remember to watch your diet and eat regular, balanced meals; avoid overeating or skipping meals; get an adequate amount of sleep; avoid alcohol, smoking or drug use (these will lower your resistance physically); and maintain some type of exercise. Exercise is one of the best ways to reduce stress. Walk with your mate, ride bikes with the children or go to the gym. This will relieve much tension.

- Add the magic. Say, "I love you," often, and be as creative as possible in conveying the message. One couple shares, "Breast cancer gave us the opportunity to fall in love all over again." Use this time as an opportunity to rekindle your relationship.

- One support partner expressed, "Today, I am a different person. I know what pain of the heart feels like, and, from knowing pain personally, I have grown into a stronger, more sensitive and compassionate person—a person I like better."

At diagnosis I thought we were given a death sentence. Today, I know that doesn't have to be the case. With the right medical team, educating yourself about cancer and faith, there can be a better quality of life after breast cancer.

Harriett now serves as a Reach To Recovery Volunteer visiting, educating and encouraging newly diagnosed patients as they begin their new battle with breast cancer. I gladly share my experiences with new support partners.

We don't take each other for granted anymore. We now have a regular habit of dating—another good thing that came out of the experience. Our relationship has priority.

—AL BARRINEAU
SUPPORT PARTNER

TAKE LIFE WITH CANCER ONE DAY AT A TIME

As you begin your journey as a support partner
For the one you love with cancer,
Take it one day at a time.

Don't spend too much time looking at the past and wondering "why,"
And don't look too far into the future asking "what."
Know that life can only be lived today.

Yesterday is history, tomorrow is the future, and
Both are out of reach.
Today is the present, and the only time you can hold on to.

When the days are emotionally tough,
Just know there are people who care about you
And are there to help.
Don't be too hard or expect too much of yourself.
Being a support partner is a new experience,
And there is much to learn.

Believe that if you take it one day at a time,
You can successfully fight your fears, self-doubt and emotional pain.
With prayer, humor, friends and your faith,
You can, as you have in the past,
Move through this problem with courage.

You can then share the courage you find with the one you love.
Together, the two of you can walk through the journey of
Breast cancer with hearts entwined,
Holding hands while sharing each other's grief.

That's what being a support partner is all about.
Just take one day at a time.

JUDY KNEECE, RN, OCN

RECOMMENDED READING

General Support

The Human Side of Cancer: Living with Hope, Coping with Uncertainty
Jimmie C. Holland, M.D.
Sheldon Lewis

Relationship Rescue
Phillip C. McGraw, Ph.D.

Sexuality and Fertility After Cancer
Leslie R. Schover, Ph.D.

Children

Talking With Kids About Cancer
Dave Dravecky, Outreach of Hope

Heaven's Not a Crying Place
Joey O'Conner

Christian Reading

The Encouragement Bible: The Answer for Those Who Hurt
New International Version
Dave Dravecky's Out Reach of Hope
David and Jan Dravecky and
Joni Eareckson Tada

Dear God, It's Cancer
William A. Fintel, M.D.
Gerald R. McDermott, Ph. D

Do Not Lose Heart
Steve Halliday

Where Is God When It Hurts?
Philip Yancey

When Life Hurts
Philip Yancey

Surprised by Suffering
R. C. Sproul

A Grace Disguised
Gerald L. Sittser

Stand By Me
Dave and Jan Dravecky

The Power of Encouragement
David Jeremiah

Hinds Feet In High Places
Hannah Hurnard

Laugh Again
Charles Swindoll

* The Encourager Magazine
www.OutreachOfHope.org

For Women

Fighting For Our Future
Beth Murphy

Thanks for the Mammogram
Laura Jansen Walker

I'm Alive and The Doctor's Dead
Sue Buchanan

You Are Not Alone - resource guide or video from the American Cancer Society

* Books can be ordered from:
   Dave Dravecky's Outreach of Hope
   719-481-3528
   www.OutreachOfHope.org

RESOURCES

General Cancer Information

American Cancer Society (ACS)
800-ACS-2345
www.cancer.org

National Cancer Institute (NCI)
800-4CANCER
www.nci.nih.gov

National Alliance of Breast Cancer Organizations (NABCO)
www.nabco.org

Susan G. Komen Foundation
800-I'M AWARE
www.komen.com

American Society of Clinical Oncology
People Living With Cancer
www.peoplelivingwithcancer.org

Information for Young Women

Young Survival Coalition
1-877-YSC-1011
www.youngsurvival.org

Support and Inspiration

Dave Dravecky's Outreach of Hope
719-481-3528
www.davedravecky.org

Stephen Ministries
(transdenominational support)
314-428-2600
www.stephenministries.com

Children's Support and Education

Kids Konnected
800-899-2866
www.kidskonnected.org

GLOSSARY

I t is important to understand the medical terminology related to your mate's diagnosis and treatments. The following is a list of the most common medical terms used in breast cancer. If you do not understand the technical language used by doctors or nurses, ask them to explain what they mean. Understanding the terms will enable you to be a more effective support partner.

A

Abscess — A collection of pus from infection.

Acini — The parts of the breast gland where fluid or milk is produced (singular: acinus).

Acute — Occurring suddenly or over a short period of time.

Adenocarcinoma — A form of cancer that involves cells from the lining of the walls of many different organs of the body. Breast cancer is a type of adenocarcinoma.

Adjuvant Treatment — Treatment that is added to increase the effectiveness of a primary treatment. In cancer, adjuvant treatment usually refers to chemotherapy, hormonal therapy, or radiation therapy after surgery to increase the likelihood of killing all cancer cells.

Alkylating Agents — A type of chemotherapy drug used in cancer treatment.

Alopecia — Refers to hair loss as a result of chemotherapy or radiation therapy administered to the head. Hair loss from chemotherapy is temporary. Hair loss from radiation is usually permanent.

Amenorrhea — The absence or discontinuation of menstrual periods.

Analgesic — Medicine given to control pain; for example: Aspirin or Tylenol®.

Anesthesia — Medication that causes entire or partial loss of feeling or sensation.

Androgen — A male sex hormone. Androgens may be used in patients with breast cancer to treat recurrence of the disease.

Aneuploid — The characteristic of having either fewer or more than the normal number of chromosomes in a cell. This is an abnormal cell.

Anorexia — Severe, uncontrolled loss of appetite.

Antiemetic — A medicine that prevents or relieves nausea and vomiting, used during and sometimes after chemotherapy.

Antimetabolites — Anti-cancer drugs that interfere with the processes of DNA production, thus preventing cell division.

Areola — The circular field of dark colored skin surrounding the nipple.

Aspiration — The procedure of removing fluid or cells from tissue by inserting a needle into an area and drawing the fluid into the syringe.

Asymptomatic — Without obvious signs or symptoms of disease. Cancer may cause symptoms and warning signs; but, especially in its early stages, it may develop and grow without producing any symptoms.

Atypical Cells — Not usual; abnormal cells. Cancer is the result of atypical cell division.

Axilla — The armpit.

Axillary Dissection — Surgical removal of lymph nodes from the armpit. This tissue is then sent to the pathologist to determine if the breast cancer has spread outside of the breast. The number of nodes removed varies during surgery. The physician can tell you how many nodes were removed.

Axillary Nodes — The lymph nodes in the axilla (underarm) that are moved and examined during surgery to see if the cancer has spread past the breast. The number of nodes in this area varies.

B

Benign Tumor — An abnormal growth that is not cancer and does not spread to other parts of the body.

Bilateral — Pertains to both sides of the body. For example, bilateral breast cancer would be on both sides of the body, or in both breasts.

Biological Response Modifier — Treatment used that alters the body's natural response to stimulate bone marrow to make specific blood cells. Referred to as colony stimulating factors.

Biopsy — The surgical removal of a small piece of tissue or a small tumor for microscopic examination to determine if cancer cells are present. A biopsy is the most important procedure in diagnosing cancer.

Biotherapy — Treatments used to stimulate the body's immune system.

Blood Count — A test from a blood sample to measure the number of red blood cells (RBCs), white blood cells (WBCs), or platelets.

Bone Marrow — The soft, fatty substance filling the cavities of the bones. Blood cells are manufactured in the bone marrow. Chemotherapy will affect the bone marrow, resulting in a temporary decrease in the number of cells in the blood.

Bone Marrow Biopsy and Aspiration — A procedure in which a needle is inserted into the center of a bone, usually the hip, to remove a small amount of bone marrow for microscopic examination.

Bone Scan — The injection of a trace amount of radioactive substance into the bloodstream to illuminate the bones under a special camera to see if the cancer has spread to the bones.

Breast Cancer — A disease of abnormal cells, with uncontrolled growth, in the breast. If not removed from the body, breast cancer has the ability to leave the breast through the lymphatic or blood systems and go to other vital organs and continue to grow. In vital distant organs, the disease can become life threatening.

Breast Implants — A round or teardrop shaped sac inserted into the body to restore the shape of the breast. May be filled with saline water or synthetic material.

Breast Self-Exam (BSE) — A procedure to examine the breast thoroughly once a month to detect any changes or suspicious lumps. Exams should be practiced at the end of the period or seven days after the start of the period. For non-menstruating women it should be performed monthly around the same time.

C

Calcifications — Small calcium deposits in breast tissue seen on mammography. The smallest object detected on mammography. May be macro (large) or micro (small) in size. Deposits are the result of cell death. Occurs with benign and malignant changes. Calcifications not caused by dietary calcium. Different shapes and patterns of occurrence give a radiologist an indication of the probable cause and whether or not biopsy is needed to evaluate calcifications.

Cancer — A general term used to describe more than 100 different uncontrolled growths of abnormal cells in the body. Cancer cells have the ability to continue to grow, invade, and destroy surrounding tissues, and leave the original site and travel via lymph or blood systems to other parts of the body where they can set up new cancerous tumors.

Cancer Cell — A cell that divides and reproduces abnormally with uncontrolled growth. This cell can break away and travel to other parts of the body and set up another site, referred to as metastasis.

Clavicle — The collarbone.

Carcinoembryonic Antigen (CEA) — Blood test used to follow women with metastatic breast cancer to help determine if the treatment is working. This is not a test specific for cancer but a marker for treatment effectiveness.

Carcinogen — Any substance that initiates or promotes the development of cancer. For example, asbestos is a proven carcinogen.

Carcinoma — A form of cancer that develops in tissues covering or lining organs of the body, such as the skin, the uterus, the lung or the breast.

Carcinoma In Situ — An early stage of development, when the cancer is still confined to the tissues of origin. It has not spread outside the area in which it began. In situ carcinomas are highly curable with surgery.

CAT Scan or CT Scan — An x-ray view of the body in sections.

Cell — The basic structural unit of all life. All living matter is composed of cells.

Cellulitis — Infection occurring in soft tissues. The surgical arm has an increased risk for cellulitis because of the removal of lymph nodes. Pain, swelling and warmth occur in the area, requiring immediate attention by a physician for an antibiotic.

Chemotherapy — Treatment of cancer by use of chemicals. Usually refers to drugs used to treat cancer.

Clinical Trial — A type of research study that tests an investigational new drug or method to see how well it works on people. The study is overseen by the Food and Drug Administration and may be carried out in a clinic or other medical facility.

Combination Chemotherapy — Treatment consisting of two or more chemicals to achieve maximum destruction of tumor cells.

Combined Modality Therapy — Two or more types of treatments used to supplement each other. For instance, surgery, radiation, chemotherapy, hormonal, or immunotherapy may be used alternatively or together for maximum effectiveness.

Complete Blood Count (CBC) — A laboratory test to determine the number of red blood cells, white blood cells, platelets, hemoglobin, and other components of a blood sample.

Computerized Tomography Scans — Commonly called CT scans. These specialized x-ray studies are used to study the internal portions of the body.

Cooper's Ligaments — Flexible bands of tissue that pass from the chest muscle between the lobes of the breasts which provide shape to and support the breasts.

Core Biopsy — Removal (with a large needle) of a piece of a lump. The sample tissue is sent to the lab to see if it is benign or malignant.

Cyst — An abnormal saclike structure that contains liquid or semisolid material. Lumps in the breast are often found to be harmless, benign cysts.

Cytology — Study of cells under a microscope that have been aspirated with a needle or scraped off organs to examine cells for signs of disease.

Cytotoxic — Drugs that can cause the death of cancer cells. Usually refers to drugs used in chemotherapy treatments.

D

Detection — The discovery of an abnormality in an asymptomatic or symptomatic person.

Diagnosis — The process of identifying a disease by its characteristic signs, symptoms and laboratory findings. With cancer, the earlier the diagnosis is made, the better the chance for a cure.

Differentiated — The similarity between a normal cell and the cancer cell; defines what degree of change has occurred. Cancer cells that are well differentiated are close to the original cell and are usually less aggressive. Poorly differentiated cells have changed more and are more aggressive.

Diploid — The characteristic of having two sets of chromosomes in a cell. This is normal for a breast cell.

DNA — One of two nucleic acids (the other is RNA) found in the nucleus of all cells. DNA contains genetic information on cell growth, division and cell function.

Doubling Time — The time required for a cell to double in number. Breast cancer has been shown to double in size every 23 to 209 days. It would take one cell, doubling every 100 days, eight to ten years to reach one centimeter or 3/8 inch in size.

Ductal Carcinoma In Situ — Cancer cells inside the ducts of a breast that have not grown through the wall of the duct into the surrounding tissues. Sometimes referred to as a pre-cancer. Prognosis is good with in situ cancers.

Ductal Papilloma — Small noncancerous finger-like growths in the mammary duct that may cause a bloody nipple discharge. Commonly found in women 45 to 50 years of age.

E

Edema — Excess fluid in the body or a body part described as swollen or puffy.

Endocrine Manipulation — Treating breast cancer by changing the hormonal balance of the body to prevent hormone-dependent cancer cells from multiplying.

Estrogen — A major female hormone secreted by the ovaries that is essential for menstruation, reproduction, and the development of secondary sex characteristics, such as breasts.

Estrogen Receptor Assay (ERA) — A test performed on cancerous tissue to see if a breast cancer is hormone-dependent and may be treated with hormonal therapy. The test reveals if cancer is estrogen receptor positive or negative. Estrogen positive cancers are often treated with hormonal therapy.

Excisional Biopsy — Surgical removal of a lump or suspicious tissue by cutting the skin and removing the tissue.

F

Familial Cancer — One occurring in families more frequently than would be expected by chance.

Fat Necrosis Tumor — A hard noncancerous lump caused by destruction of fat cells in the breast due to trauma or injury.

Fibroadenoma — A noncancerous, solid tumor most commonly found in younger women.

Fibrocystic Breast Changes or Condition — A noncancerous breast condition in which multiple cysts or lumpy areas develop in one or both breasts. It can be accompanied by discomfort or pain that fluctuates with the menstrual cycle. Large cysts can be treated by aspiration of the fluid they contain.

Fine Needle Aspiration — Procedure to remove cells or fluid from tissues using a needle with an empty syringe. Cells or breast fluid are extracted by pulling back on plunger and are then analyzed by a physician.

Flow Cytometry — A test done on cancerous tissues that shows the aggressiveness of the tumor. It shows how many cells are in the dividing stage at one time, commonly referred to as the 'S' phase, and the DNA content of the cancer, referred to as the 'ploidy'. This reveals how rapidly the tumor is growing.

Frozen Section — A technique in which a part of the biopsy tissue is frozen immediately, and a thin slice is then mounted on a microscope slide, enabling a pathologist to analyze it in just a few minutes for a diagnosis.

Frozen Shoulder — Surgical shoulder which has severely restricted range of motion and is painful.

G

Galactocele – A clogged milk duct that occurs in breastfeeding women. Similar to a cyst, but filled with milk.

Genes — Located in the nucleus of the cell, genes contain hereditary information that is transferred from cell to cell.

Genetic — Refers to the inherited pattern located in genes for certain characteristics.

H

Hematoma — A collection of blood that can form in a wound after surgery, or aspiration, or can be caused from an injury.

Hormonal Therapy — Treatment of cancer by alteration of the hormonal balance. Some cancer will only grow in the presence of certain hormones.

Hormone — Secreted by various organs in the body, hormones help regulate growth, metabolism and reproduction. Some hormones are used as treatment following surgery for breast, ovarian and prostate cancers.

Hormone Receptor Assay — A diagnostic test to determine whether hormones influence a breast cancer's growth and also determines whether or not it can be treated with hormones.

Hot Flashes — A sensation of heat and flushing that occurs suddenly. May be associated with menopause or some medications.

Hyperplasia — An abnormal, excessive growth of cells that is benign.

I

Intramuscular (I.M.) — To receive a medication by needle injection into a muscle of the body.

Immune System — Complex system by which the body protects itself from outside invaders that are harmful to the body.

Immunology — Study of the body's mechanisms of resistance against disease or invasion by foreign substances. The ability of the body to fight a disease.

Immunotherapy — A treatment that stimulates the body's own defense mechanisms to combat diseases such as cancer.

Immunosuppressed — Condition of having a lowered resistance to disease. May be a temporary result of lowered white blood cells from chemotherapy administration.

Incisional Biopsy — A surgical incision made through the skin to remove a portion of a suspected lump or tissue.

Inflammation — Reaction of tissue to various conditions that may result in pain, redness, or warmth of tissues in the area.

Infiltrating (Invasive) Cancer — Cancer that has grown through the cell wall of the breast area, in which it originated, and into surrounding tissues.

Informed Consent — Process of explanation to the patient of all risks and complications of a procedure or treatment before it is done. Most informed consents are written and signed by the patient or a legal representative.

Intraductal — Residing within the duct of the breast. Intraductal disease may be benign or malignant.

Invasive Cancer — Cancer that has spread outside its site of origin and is growing into the surrounding tissues.

In Situ — In place, localized and confined to one area. Cancer that has not grown through the cell wall of where it began. A very early stage of cancer.

Infiltrating Ductal Cell Carcinoma — A cancer that starts in the mammary glands and has spread to areas outside the gland.

Intravenous (I.V.) — Entering the body through a vein.

Inverted Nipple — The turning inward of the nipple. Usually a congenital condition; but, if it occurs where it has not previously existed, it can be a sign of benign or malignant disease.

L

Lactation — Process of milk production from the breasts.

Lesion — An area of tissue that is diseased, may be benign or malignant.

Leukocyte — A white blood cell or corpuscle that fights infection in the body.

Leukopenia — A decrease in the number of white blood cells resulting in susceptibility to infection.

Linear Accelerator — A machine that produces high-energy x-ray beams to destroy cancer cells.

Liver Scan — A way of visualizing the liver by injecting into the bloodstream a trace dose of a radioactive substance which helps visualize the organ during x-ray.

Lobular — Pertaining to the part of the breast that is furthest from the nipple, the part of the lobes where milk is produced.

Localized Cancer — A cancer still confined to its site of origin.

Lump — Any kind of abnormal mass in the breast or elsewhere in the body.

Lumpectomy — A surgical procedure in which only the cancerous tumor and an area of surrounding tissue is removed. Usually the surgeon will remove some of the underarm lymph nodes or perform a sentinel node biopsy at the same time. This procedure is also referred to as a tylectomy.

Lymphatic Vessels — Vessels that remove cellular waste from the body by filtering through lymph nodes and eventually emptying into the vascular (blood) system.

Lymph — A clear fluid circulating throughout the body in the lymphatic system that contains white blood cells and antibodies.

Lymph Gland — Also called a lymph node. These are rounded tissues in the lymphatic system that vary in size from a pinhead to an olive and may appear in groups or one at a time. The principal ones are in the neck, underarm and groin. These glands produce lymphocytes and monocytes (white blood cells which fight foreign substances) and serve as filters to prevent bacteria from entering the bloodstream. They will filter out cancer cells but can also serve as a site for metastatic disease. The major ones serving the breast are in the armpit. Some are located above and below the collarbone and some in between the ribs near the breastbone. There are three levels of lymph nodes in the underarm area of the breast and another around the breastbone. Number of nodes vary from person to person. Lymph nodes are usually sampled during surgery to determine if the cancer has spread outside of the breast area.

Lymphedema — A swelling in the arm caused by excess fluid that collects after the lymph nodes have been removed by surgery or affected by radiation treatments.

M

Macrocyst — A cyst that is large enough to be felt with the fingers.

Magnification View — Special enlarged views used in mammography to magnify an area for greater detail of suspicious finding.

Magnetic Resonance Imaging (MRI) — A magnet scan; a form of x-ray using magnets instead of radiation. MRI gives a more clearly defined picture of fatty tissue than x-ray.

Malignant Tumor — A mass of cancer cells. These cells have uncontrolled growth and will invade surrounding tissues and spread to distant sites of the body setting up new cancer sites, a process called metastasis.

Mammary Duct Ectasia — A noncancerous breast disease most often found in women during menopause. The ducts in or beneath the nipple become clogged with cellular and fatty debris. The duct may have gray to greenish discharge, a lump that can be felt, and can become inflamed, causing pain.

Mammary Glands — The breast glands that produce and carry milk by way of the mammary ducts to the nipples during pregnancy and breastfeeding.

Mammogram — An x-ray of the breast that can detect tumors before they can be felt. A baseline mammogram is performed on healthy breasts, usually at the age of 35, to establish a basis for later comparison.

Mammotest — Biopsy performed under mammography while breast is compressed and lesion is viewed by physician. Sample of lesion is removed using a large core needle and is then sent to lab to determine if it is benign or malignant.

Margins — The area of tissue surrounding a tumor when it is removed by surgery.

Mastalgia — Pain occurring in the breast.

Mastectomy — Surgical removal of the breast and some of the surrounding tissue.

Radical Mastectomy — The most common type of mastectomy. Breast skin, nipple, areola and underarm lymph   nodes are removed. The chest muscles are saved.

Prophylactic Mastectomy — A procedure sometimes recommended for patients at a very high risk for developing cancer in one or both sides.

Subcutaneous mastectomy — Performed before cancer is detected, removes the breast tissue but leaves the outer skin, areola and nipple intact. (This is not suitable with a diagnosis of cancer.)

Radical Mastectomy (Halsted Radical) — The surgical removal of the breast, breast skin, nipple, areola, chest muscles, and underarm lymph nodes.

Segmental Mastectomy (Partial Mastectomy/ Lumpectomy) — A surgical procedure in which only a portion of the breast is removed, including the cancer and the surrounding margin of healthy breast tissue.

Mastitis — Infection occurring in the breast. Pain, tenderness, swelling, redness, and warmth occurs in one quadrant of the breast and spreads quickly. Infection requires antibiotics.

Menopause — The time in a woman's life when the menstrual cycle ends and the ovaries produce lower levels of hormones; usually occurs between the age of 45 and 55.

Metastasis — The spread of cancer from one part of the body to another through the lymphatic system or the bloodstream. The cells in the new cancer location are the same type as those in the original sites.

Microcalcifications — Particles observed on a mammogram that are found in the breast tissue appearing as small spots on the picture. Usually occur from calcium deposits caused by death of breast cells which may be benign or malignant. When clustered in one area, may need to be checked more closely for a malignant change in the breast.

Microcyst — A cyst that is too small to be felt but may be observed on mammography or ultrasound screening.

Micrometastasis — Undetectable spread of cancer outside of the breast that is not seen on routine screening tests. Metastasis is too limited to have created enough mass to be observed.

Multicentric — More than one origin or place of growth in the breast. These growths may or may not be related to each other.

Myleosuppression — A decrease in the ability of the bone marrow cells to produce blood cells, including red blood cells, white blood cells, and platelets. This condition increases susceptibility to infection and produces fatigue.

N

Needle Biopsy — Removal of a sample of tissue from the breast using a wide-core needle with suction.

Necrosis — Death of a tissue.

Neoplasm — Any abnormal growth. Neoplasms may be benign or malignant, but the term is usually used to describe a cancer.

Nodularity — Increased density of breast tissue, most often due to hormonal changes in the breast, which causes the breast to feel lumpy in texture. This finding is called normal nodularity, and it usually occurs in both breasts.

Nodule — A small, solid mass.

Oncogene — Certain stretches of cellular DNA. Genes that, when inappropriately activated, contribute to the malignant transformation of a cell.

Oncologist — A physician who specializes in cancer treatment.

Oncology — The science dealing with the physical, chemical, and biological properties and features of cancer, including causes, the disease process and therapies.

One-Step Procedure — A procedure in which a surgical biopsy is performed under general anesthesia, and if cancer is found, a mastectomy or lumpectomy is done immediately as part of the same operation.

Oophorectomy — The surgical removal of the ovaries, sometimes performed as a part of hormone therapy.

Orgasm — A state of physical and emotional excitement that occurs at the climax of sexual intercourse. In the male it is evidenced by ejaculation of semen.

Osteoporosis — Softening of bones that occurs with age, calcium loss and hormone depletion.

P

Per Orally (P.O.) — To take a medication by mouth.

Palliative Treatment — Therapy that relieves symptoms, such as pain or pressure, but does not alter the development of the disease. Its primary purpose is to improve the quality of life.

Palpation — A procedure using the hands to examine organs such as the breast. A palpable mass is one you can feel with your hands.

Pathology — The study of disease through the microscopic examination of body tissues and organs. Any tumor suspected of being cancerous must be diagnosed by pathological examination.

Pathologist — A physician with special training in diagnosing diseases from samples of tissue.

Pectoralis Muscles — Muscular tissues attached to the front of the chest wall and extending to the upper arms. These are under the breast. They are divided into the pectoralis major and the pectoralis minor muscles.

Permanent Section — A technique in which a thin slice of biopsy tissue is mounted on a slide to be examined under a microscope by a pathologist in order to establish a diagnosis.

Platelet — A cell formed by the bone marrow and circulating in the blood that is necessary for blood clotting. Platelet transfusions are used in cancer patients to prevent or control bleeding when the number of platelets have decreased.

Ploidy — The number of chromosome sets in a cell.

Port, Life Port, Port-A-Cath — A device surgically implanted under the skin, usually on the chest, that enters a large blood vessel and is used to deliver medication, chemotherapy, blood products and also is used to obtain blood samples. A port is usually inserted if a person has veins in the arm which are difficult to use for treatment or if certain types of chemotherapy drugs are to be given.

Precancerous — Abnormal cellular changes that are potentially capable of becoming cancer. These early lesions are very amenable to treatment and cure. Also called pre-malignant.

Progesterone — Female hormone produced by the ovaries during a specific time in the menstrual cycle. Causes the uterus to prepare for pregnancy and the breasts to get ready to produce milk.

Progesterone Receptor Assay (PRA) — A test that is done on cancerous tissue to see if a breast cancer is hormone (progesterone) dependent and can be treated by hormonal therapy.

Prognosis — A prediction of the course of the disease—the future prospect for the patient. For example, most breast cancer patients who receive treatment early have a good prognosis.

Prolactin — Female hormone which stimulates the development of the breast and later is essential for starting and continuing milk production.

Prophylactic Mastectomy — Removal of high-risk breast tissue to prevent future development of cancer.

Prosthesis — An artificial form. In the case of breast cancer following mastectomy, a breast form that can be worn inside a bra.

Protocol — A schedule of selected drugs and treatment time intervals known to be effective against a certain cancer.

R

Radiation Therapy — Treatment with high energy x-rays to destroy cancer cells.

Radiation Oncologist — A physician specifically trained in the use of high energy x-rays to treat cancer.

Radiologist — A physician who specializes in diagnoses of diseases by the use of x-rays.

Radiotherapy — Treatment of cancer with high energy radiation. Radiation therapy may be used to reduce the size of a cancer before surgery or to destroy any remaining cancer cells after surgery. Radiotherapy can be helpful in shrinking recurrent cancer to relieve symptoms such as pain and pressure.

Recurrence — Reappearance of cancer after a period of remission.

Regional Involvement — The spread of cancer from its original site to nearby surrounding areas. Regional cancers are confined to one location of the body. Regional involvement in breast cancer could include spread to the lymph nodes or to the chest wall.

Rehabilitation — Programs that help patients adjust and return to full productive lives. May involve physical therapy, the use of a prosthesis, and counseling and emotional support.

Relapse — The reappearance of cancer after a disease-free period.

Remission — Complete or partial disappearance of the signs and symptoms of disease in response to treatment. The period during which a disease is under control. A remission, however, is not necessarily a cure.

Retraction — Process of skin pulling in toward breast tissue. Often referred to as dimpling.

Risk Factors — Anything that increases an individual's chance of getting a disease such as cancer. The risk factors for breast disease are a first degree relative with breast cancer, a high fat diet, early menstruation, late menopause, first child after 30 or no children.

Risk Reduction — Techniques used to reduce chances of getting a certain cancer. For example, reducing dietary fat may help prevent breast cancer.

S

S Phase — Test that is performed to determine how many cells within the tumor are in a stage of division.

Sarcoma — A form of cancer that arises in the supportive tissues such as bone, cartilage, fat or muscle.

Secondary Tumor — A tumor that develops as a result of metastasis or spreads beyond the original cancer.

Secondary Site — A second site in which cancer is found. Example: cancer in the lymph nodes near the breast is a secondary site.

Side Effects — Usually describes situations that occur after treatments. For example, hair loss may be a side effect of chemotherapy, or fatigue may be a side effect of radiation therapy.

Staging — An evaluation of the extent of a disease, such as breast cancer. A classification based on stage at diagnosis which helps determine the appropriate treatment and prognosis. In breast cancer, it is determined by whether the lymph nodes are involved; if the cancer has spread to other parts of the body (through the lymphatic system or bloodstream) and set up distant metastasis; and the size of tumor. Five different stages are used in breast cancer with levels in each stage. Stage IV is the most serious.

Stellate — Appearing on mammography as a starshape because of the irregular growth of cells into surrounding tissue. May be associated with a malignancy or some benign conditions.

Stereotactic Needle Biopsy — Biopsy done while breast is compressed under mammography. A series of pictures locate the lesion, and a radiologist enters information into a computer. The computer calculates information and positions a needle to remove the finding. A needle is inserted into the lump, and a piece of tissue is removed and sent to the lab for analysis. May be referred to as mammotest or core biopsy.

Stomatitis — Inflammation of the gastrointestinal tract creating discomfort and a potential for infection. May be caused by chemotherapy drugs.

Supraclavicular Nodes — The nodes located above the collarbone in the area of the neck.

T

Tamoxifen — (Nolvadex®) An antiestrogen, nonsteroidal drug that may be given to breast cancer patients to block the effects of estrogen on breast tissues, reducing the risk of recurrence. The most common side effects reported are hot flashes, vaginal discharge and menstrual irregularities.

Thrombocytopenia — A decrease in the number of platelets in the blood resulting in the potential for increased bleeding and decreased ability for clotting.

Tissue — A collection of similar cells. There are four basic types of tissues in the body: epithelial, connective, muscle, and nerve.

Tumor — An abnormal tissue, swelling or mass, may be either benign or malignant.

Two-Step Procedure — When surgical biopsy and breast surgery are performed in two separate surgeries.

U

Ultrasound Examination — The use of high frequency sound waves to locate a tumor inside the body. Helps determine if a breast lump is solid tissue or filled with fluids.

Ultrasound Guided Biopsy — The use of ultrasound to guide a biopsy needle to obtain a sample of tissue for analysis by a pathologist.

REFERENCES

Bennett B.B., Steinbach B.G, Hardt N.S., and Haigh L.S., *Breast Disease for Clinicians*, New York, NY: McGraw Hill, 2001

Dixon J.M. and Morrow M., *Breast Disease: A Problem-Based Approach*. New York: W.B. Saunders, 1999

Holland, J. C., Lewis, S. *The Human Side of Cancer*, Harper Collins Publishers, 2000

Holland, J. C., *Psycho-oncology*, New York: Oxford University Press, 1998

Hudson, Tori, *Women's Encyclopedia of Natural Medicine*. Los Angeles, CA: Keats Publishing, 1999

Hughes L.E., Mansel R.E., and Webster D.J.T., *Benign Disorders and Diseases of the Breast*. Philadelphia, PA: W.B. Saunders, 2000

Hunt K.K., Robb G.L, Strom E.A., and Ueno N.T. *Breast Cancer* (M.D. Anderson Cancer Series). New York, NY: Springer-Verlag, 2001

Lippman M.E., Morrow M., Hellman S., and Harris J.R., *Diseases of the Breast*. Philadelphia, PA: Lippincott-Raven, 1996.

Marchant D.J., *Contemporary Management of Breast Diseases: Benign Disease*. Philadelphia, PA: W. B. Saunders, 1994.

Pazdur R., Coia L.R., Hoskins W.J., and Wagman L.D., *Cancer Management: A Multidisciplinary Approach*. Melville, NY: PRR, 2002

Physicians Desk Reference, Breast Cancer Disease Management, Montvale, NJ: Medical Economics Company, Inc. 2002

Schover, L. R., *Sexuality and Fertility After Cancer*: John Wiley & Sons, Inc. 1997

Silva O.E. and Zurrida S., *Breast Cancer: A Practical Guide*, New York, NY: Elsevier Science Ltd., 2000

Simon, J., Houston, V., *Restore Yourself*, New York: Berkley Books, 2001

Spratt J.S. and Donegan W.L., *Cancer of the Breast*. Philadelphia, PA: W.B. Saunders Company, 1995.